LAND OF NUTRITION

FOOD IS MY RELIGION

A HEALTHY GUIDE TO WORSHIPING FOOD

Lara J McKenna

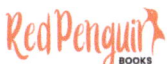

Food is My Religion

Copyright ©2025
by Lara J McKenna

ISBN
Digital 978-1-63777-765-7
Print 978-1-63777-766-4
Library of Congress Control Number: 2025917862

All rights reserved. No part of this book may be reproduced in any form or by any electronic or mechanical means, including information storage and retrieval systems, without permission in writing from the author.

Published by **Red Penguin Books**
Bellerose Village, New York

For information, contact Lara at www.LandofNutrition.com.

The content of this book is for general informational purposes only. It is not meant to be used, nor should it be used, to diagnose or treat any medical condition or to replace the services of your physician or other healthcare provider. The advice and strategies contained in the book may not be suitable for all readers. Please consult your healthcare provider for any questions that you may have about your own medical situation. Neither the author, publisher, The Institute of Integrative Nutrition (IIN) nor any of their employees or representatives guarantees the accuracy of information in this book or its usefulness to a particular reader, nor are they responsible for any damage or negative consequence that may result from any treatment, action taken or inaction by any person reading or following the information in this book.

Dedication

To my family:
Having them around the table is my biggest joy!

xoxo

Table Of Contents

FOOD IS MY RELIGION PART 1 1

INTRODUCTION: MY STORY, FOOD AND RELIGION. 3

FOOD AND RELIGION. 9

THE YES LIST 15

THE NAUGHTY LIST - INGREDIENTS TO AVOID 52

RITUALS 75

HERBAL TEA 76

BLESS YOUR MEALS AND FOOD 77

AFFIRMATIONS. 79

THE KITCHEN IS MY TEMPLE 83

THE GOLDEN RULE 87

MEAL PLANNING 90

CELEBRATE FOOD EVERYDAY. 93

WRAPPING IT UP WITH GRATITUDE 106

THE 10 COMMANDMENTS OF FOOD IS MY RELIGION 107

FOOD IS MY RELIGION PART 2 RECIPES 111

SALADS, DRESSINGS, SAUCES AND DIPS 113

Land of Nutrition Everyday Homemade Salad Dressing 113

Baby Greens Salad 113

Concord Salad 114

Caesar Salad from the Cape 115

Summer Salad 116

Yummy Kale Salad !!! 117

Christmas Salad (and our traditional Christmas meal) 118

Carrot Ginger Dressing (dip) 119

All in one Asian Dressing / Dip / Marinade	120
Chimichurri	121
Taco Seasoning	122
Mango Salsa	123
Homemade Tzatziki	124
Cucumber Tomato Salad	124

SOUPS AND STEWS 125

Gazpacho	125
Chili - 3 Ways	126
Butternut Squash Soup	127
Ramen (Radish noodle soup)	128
Uncle Stu's Chicken Noodle Soup	130

MAIN COURSES 132

Baked Chicken Cutlets	132
OKAL Chicken Marinade	133
Roasted Lemon Chicken Thighs and Cauliflower	135
Mediterranean Meatballs	136
Skirt Steak Marinade	137
Spring Vegetable Frittata	138
Baby Lamb Chop Dry-ish Marinade - Easter App or Charmed Life Tailgating	140
Grass Fed Beef Burgers	142
Hot Dogs	142
Fresh Striped Bass Ceviche	144
TNT Fish Taco	145
Cape Cod Cod	146
Holiday Brisket	148

ON THE SIDE - SIDE DISHES 149

Caramelized Onion	149

Quick Pickled Onions 150
Sauteed Green Beans 151
Homemade Sauerkraut 152
French Fries aka Roasted Potatoes 154
Yellow Rice 155
Best Potato Latkes 156
Baked Plantains 158

BAKING IS FUN, ADD SOMETHING SWEET 159
Antioxidant Truffles 159
Fool Proof Irish Soda Bread 160
Coconut Macaroons 161
Land of Nutrition Granola 162
Berry Nice Board 164
Sweet Potato Brownies 165
Heart Healthy Linzer Tarts with Chia Seed Jam 166
Zucchini Muffins 168
Lara's Almond Butter Chunks 170
Tahini Squares 171
Banana Bread 172

ELIXIRS 173
Magic Morning Tonic 173
Night Time Cherry Juice Mocktail 174

THANKSGIVING MENU 175

REFERENCE GUIDE 181
ACKNOWLEDGMENT 184
RECIPE INDEX 185

Food is My Religion

Part 1

"The First Wealth is Health"
–Ralph Waldo Emmerson

INTRODUCTION: MY STORY, FOOD AND RELIGION

Food is my religion. To begin, I respect and honor all religions in this beautiful world. I was raised in a loving Jewish home and honor my Jewish heritage and culture. I have a very healthy interfaith marriage, my husband is Catholic and I honor his beliefs and his family culture. We have raised three beautiful children, now adults, in a multifaith household, celebrated all holidays and each have our own unique beliefs and spirituality. Religion serves a big purpose in life for many people, explaining the unexplainable. I have worked and lived in spaces with a diverse group of amazing people and have learned much about religions. It is primary that religious culture brings family and friends together, the truth is- our lives REVOLVE AROUND FOOD.

With **Food is My Religion**, I will share how food is the center of my very being. And how you can live a healthy food-centric life with a few tips and tricks that I've learned around the way. It's when we know why and why not to eat certain things we are more likely to understand and stick with it.

From the moment I wake up, food occupies my attention. FOOD is what I breathe for and love to share. My kitchen is my temple, and I spend most of my days preparing, researching healthy recipes, and creating healthy meals, for myself, my family and guests. Hearing stories of favorite meals on vacations, holidays and sharing how to create everyday healthy foods, to the point of growing my own vegetables are all my favorite activities.

It is significant to note that spiritual practices often revolve around food, satiating our bodies, hearts and souls. Washing lettuce and chopping broccoli, if done with loving intention, can transform the way you eat and more importantly your health. My hope is that this book inspires and guides you to a conscious relationship with food. You will also find ideas and reflections to support your overall wellbeing. Nutrition is much more than what's on your plate.

Remember that health is wealth, you have the power to make a difference.

WHERE IT ALL BEGAN

My story is unremarkable. I was raised in the Bronx, NY, until my family moved out to the suburbs of Long Island, NY. We had family dinners most nights, since my mom always cooked from scratch, and still does. We rarely went out to dinner or ordered in. (Maybe that's why I love home cooking, and also why I appreciate a good restaurant meal.) My parents certainly did not make me eat my vegetables, and in fact, in the 70's when salt and fat were "bad," margarine was king, and no salt potato chips and pretzels were my treat. My two younger brothers and I fairly traded our pasta for meat in baked ziti and would fight over the last cookie.

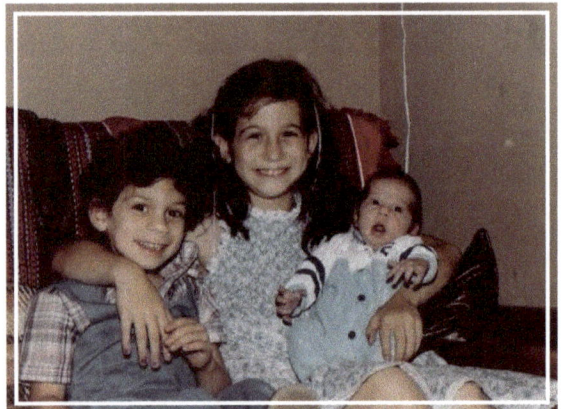
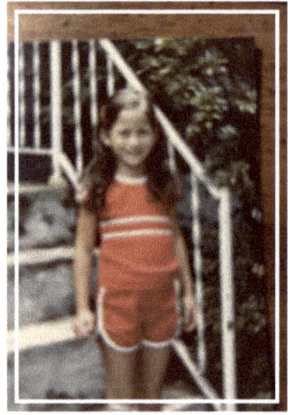
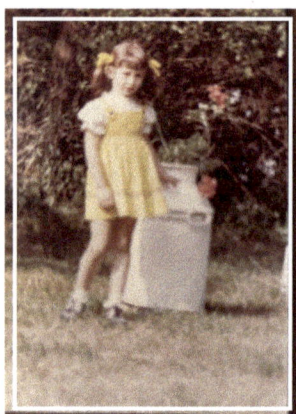

College life in upstate NY revolved around Buffalo wings, pizza, and beer. What I appreciate now is that region of New York is host to some of the best apple orchards in the world! There's nothing like a fresh New York apple - right from the tree! New York City is called The Big Apple after all.

It was at a college party one night, I looked across the room and everything in my vision went black and white, except for a very cute, familiar guy across the room, who was in full color - I knew I had to meet him! It was love at first sight. After more than two decades of being happily married, we are what some consider, an anomaly, a story for another book perhaps?

Because of our different faiths, the path was not, and still not, always easy. However, there is hope. You can break religious direction and have a healthy, thriving, wonderful interfaith relationship.

Bill and I attended an Interfaith Pre-Cana, in the year 2000, a catholic tradition that before a couple weds they spend some time with each other in a classroom-like setting, with other couples learning how to enter this new phase of union. In fact, the word Pre-Cana derives from the location of a wedding ceremony where Jesus turned water to wine. The point is to engage in "must have" conversations, basically real-life planning sessions. It can get deep, our Pre-Cana was a supportive mix of interfaith couples and it was great to get that kind of support.

In today's day and age, it is more common for a couple to fall in love with, and marry someone of a different faith, different color or same sex. We're all in this together – "Love is My Religion" - thank you Bob Marley. At the end of each session, we ate snacks and drank wine.

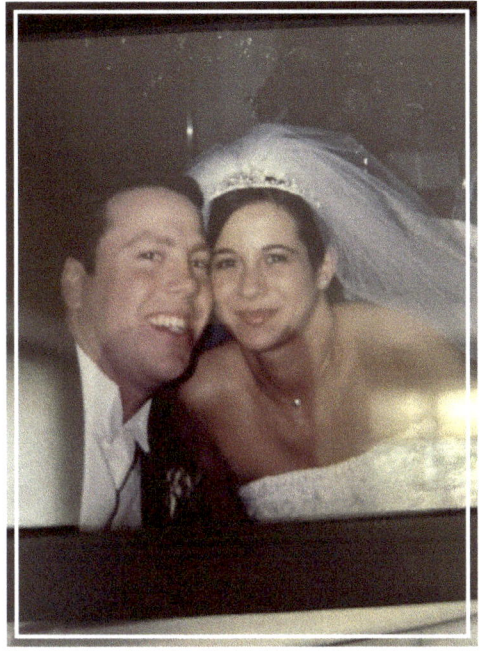

The wedding itself is a feast gathered by your closest family and friends. Or - if you favor, a secret ceremony at town hall, but I bet there is a chosen meal in there somewhere.

Life gets better. For years, I worked to lose weight after I had a baby. And then, less than two years later, I had twins - the stresses of life with three small kids was managed with a shift in my nutrition. When the shift happened, I turned to apples and herbal tea, instead of chips, candy and diet soda, and things became easier. I became stronger, more patient, less stressed and happier - I learned by trial and error how to cook in a healthy way that also tastes good!

I realized deeper that what I was eating and my nutrition had a huge effect on my life! Some simple changes made me feel so good that I just want to share it with others. Becoming a Certified Integrative Nutrition Health Coach helped me get some insights for my own wellbeing, as well as for my family and friends. I finished Institute of Integrative Nutrition in 2018 and launched LAND

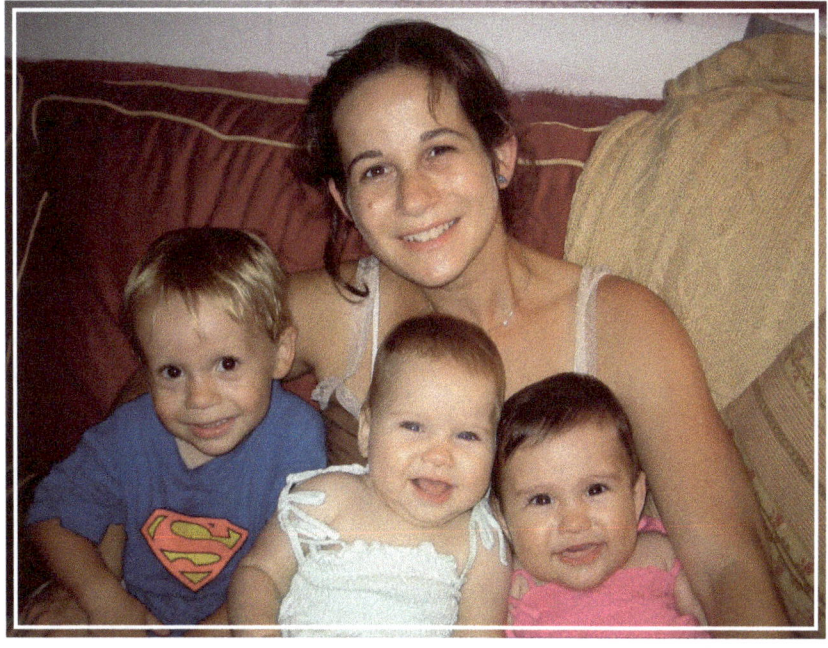

OF NUTRITION, Inc., a small business bringing health-full recipes, health ideas, coaching and support. I guide individuals and groups towards healthy habits, give healthy cooking classes, grocery tours, pantry makeovers, share recipes and teach how easy it is to grow organic veggies in my very own garden.

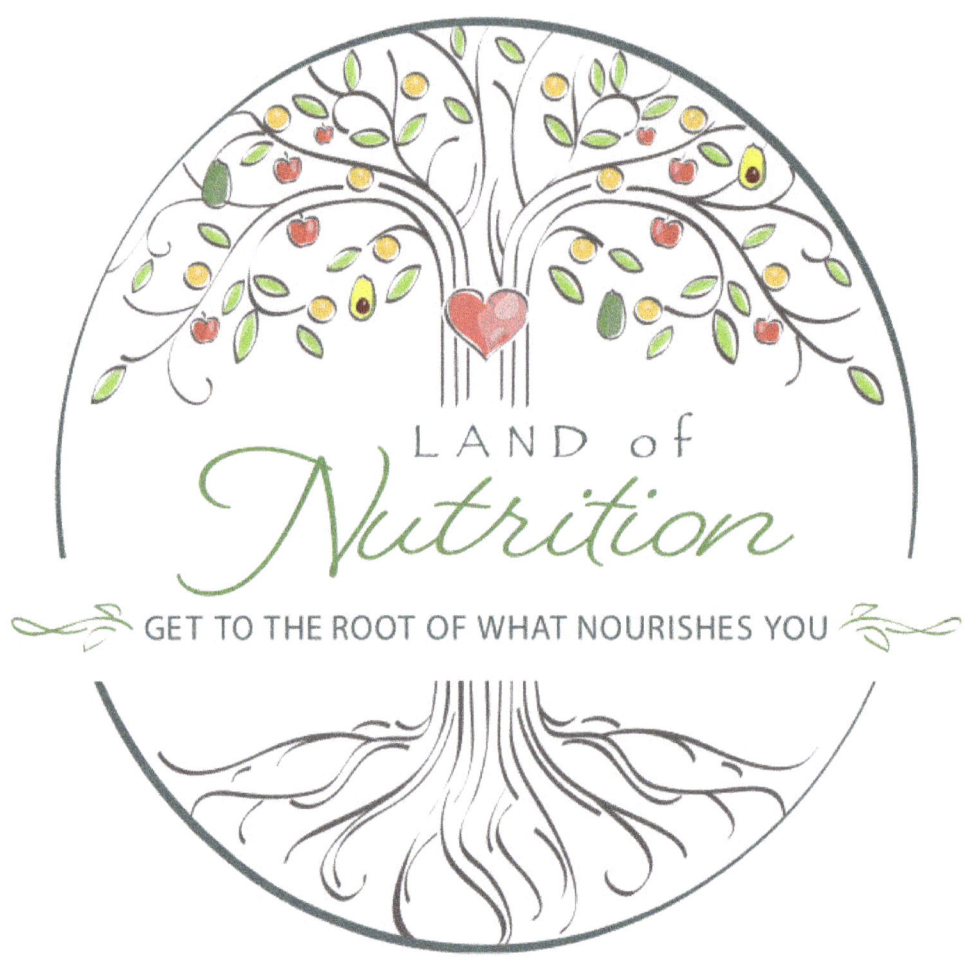

This insight of experience casts me into the role of a health and happiness advocate. Nutrition is not just what you put in your mouth, health encompasses so much more: Your emotional and physical wellbeing, quality of your relationships, sleep habits, proper nutrition, and spirituality all contribute to your health.

What we eat, how we move, how we handle stress, and what toxins we are exposed to have a huge impact on your body and brain. This is where FOOD IS MY RELIGION comes in.

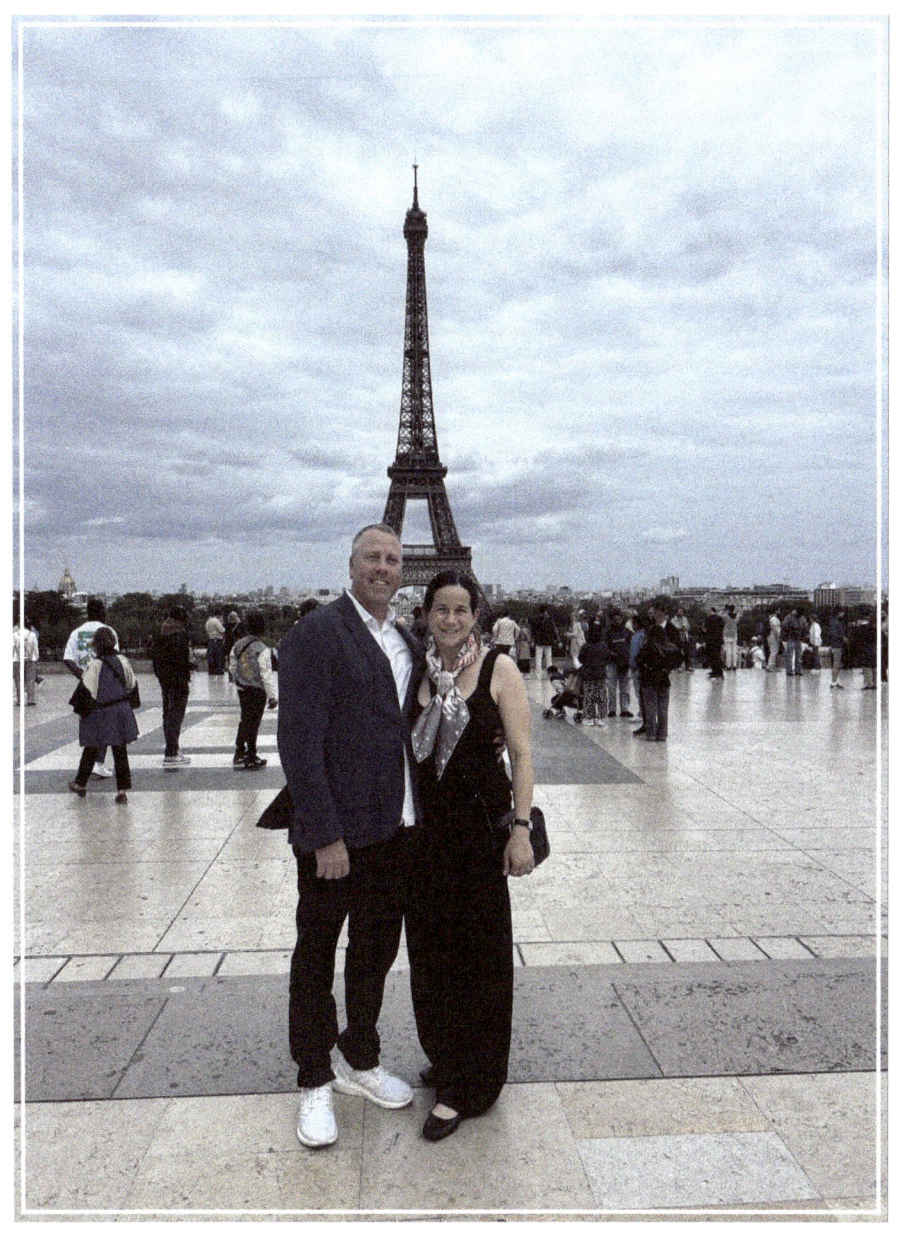

Family recipes root us, while travel expands us.
Sharing meals across cultures teaches us that food
is more than fuel—it is memory, celebration,
and love in its most universal form.

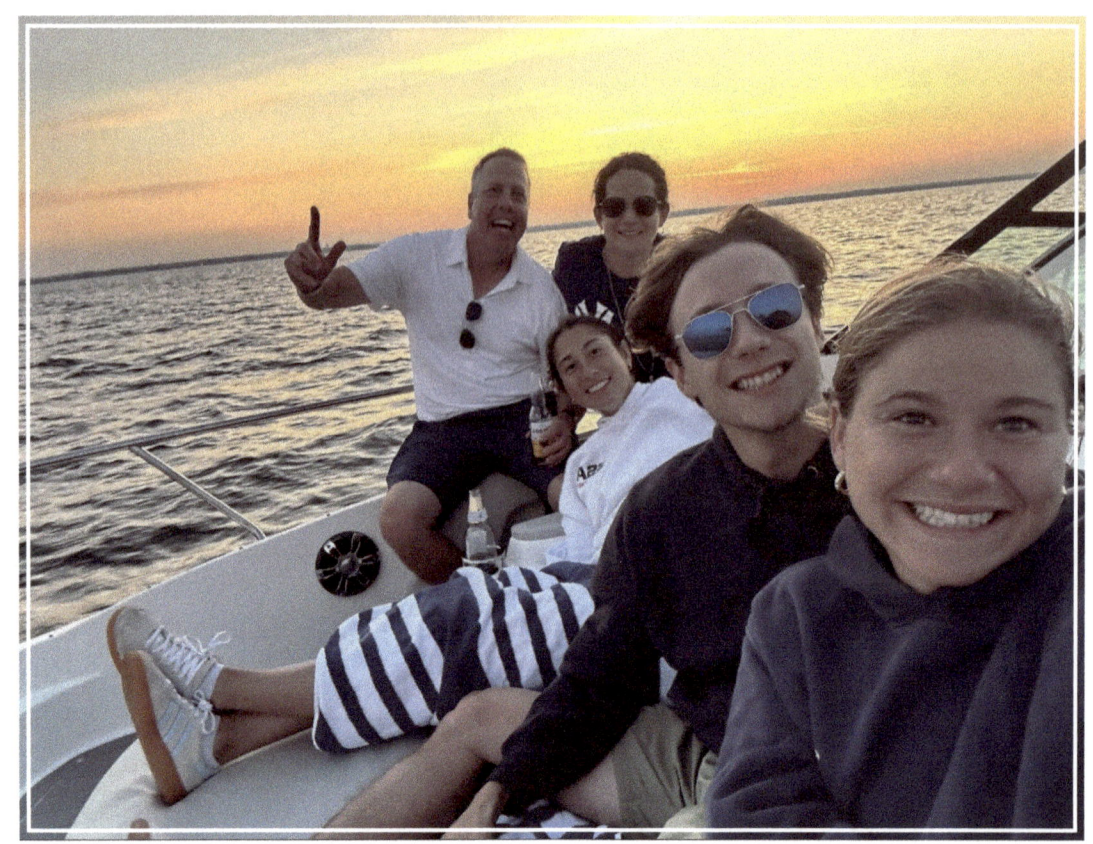

Family and food are inseparable threads in the fabric of our lives. A simple meal can carry the weight of tradition, memory, and love. As Julia Child once said, "People who love to eat are always the best people." Around the table, we find not just nourishment, but laughter, connection, and the reminder that we belong to one another. Every recipe becomes a story, and every gathering a chance to write a new chapter together.

FOOD AND RELIGION

From Apples and Honey on Rosh Hashanah (the Jewish New Year), Hot Cross Buns on Easter (the commemorating the resurrection of Jesus), to Vasilopita (a greek orthodox bread made for New Year's Day), and everything in between, I think we can all agree that religions and cultures, in general, have a lot to do with food.

When we come together with family, friends, and congregations, there is food. It starts as snack time in preschool, a time where kids can take a break, get some nourishment (we hope), laugh and have fun. We go to restaurants to meet our friends for dinner, we hold dinner parties, we meet for brunch, we celebrate birthdays, anniversaries, graduations, births, deaths, you name it, we meet for a meal.

Religion adds structure to communities. With Food Is My Religion, my intent is to add some structure to your health by way of simple concepts around nutrition, along with some fun ways to celebrate food. Today we know more about science, big bang theories and evolution than a woman taking a bite of a forbidden apple. Now, the focus can shift to protecting our health, our children's well-being, and the health of the planet we call home.

When we embrace nutrition and food in a fun loving, not an "UGH, another diet" way it is easier to fall in love with making yourself healthy and happy.

YOU REALLY ARE WHAT YOU EAT and with *Food is My Religion*, simple changes can help anyone have more energy, be happier, sleep better, that is my mission. I believe it is small intentional changes that add up to a healthier lifestyle.

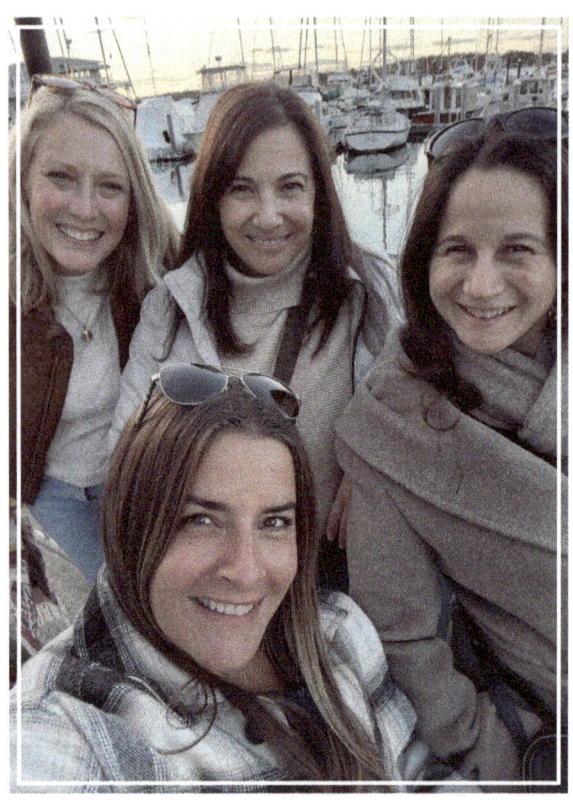
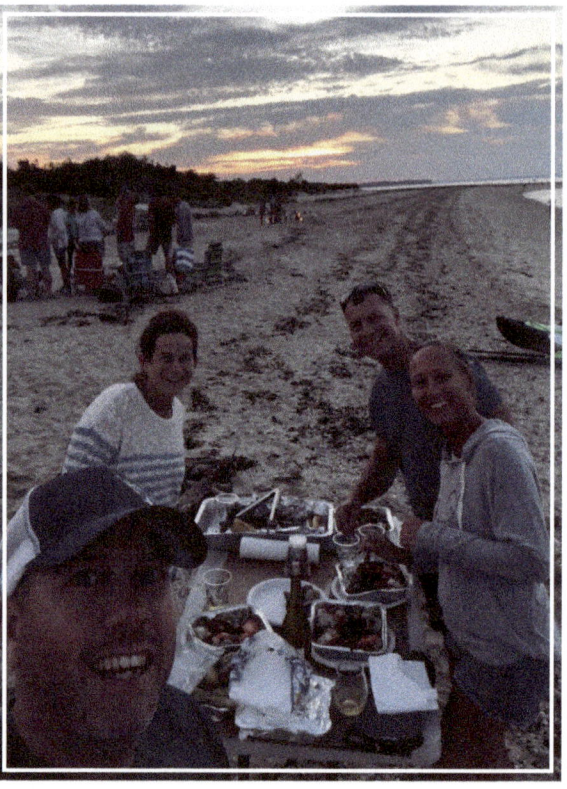
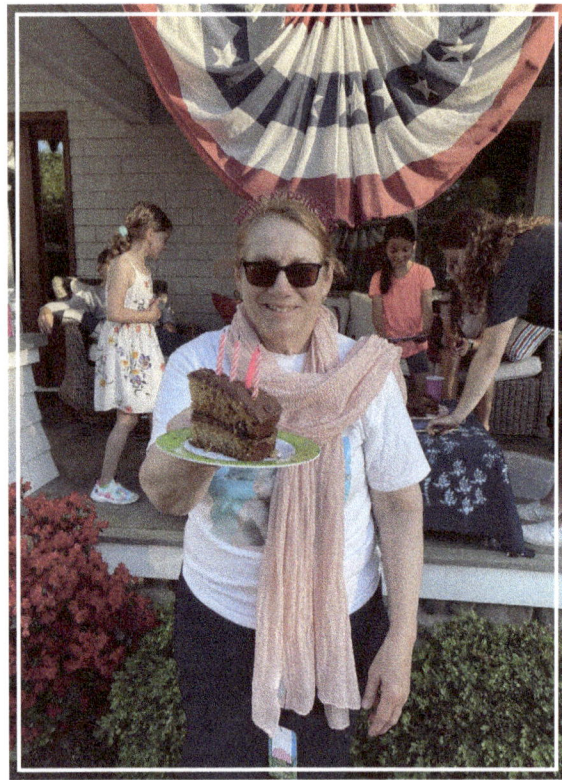
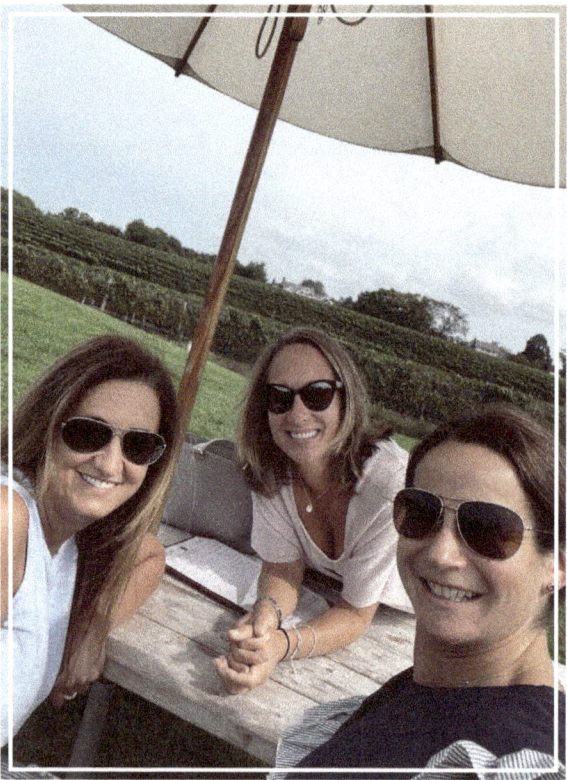

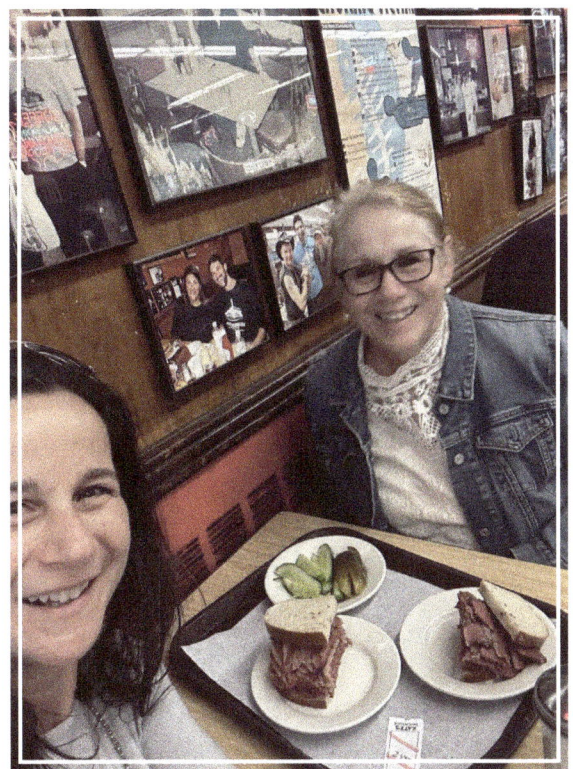
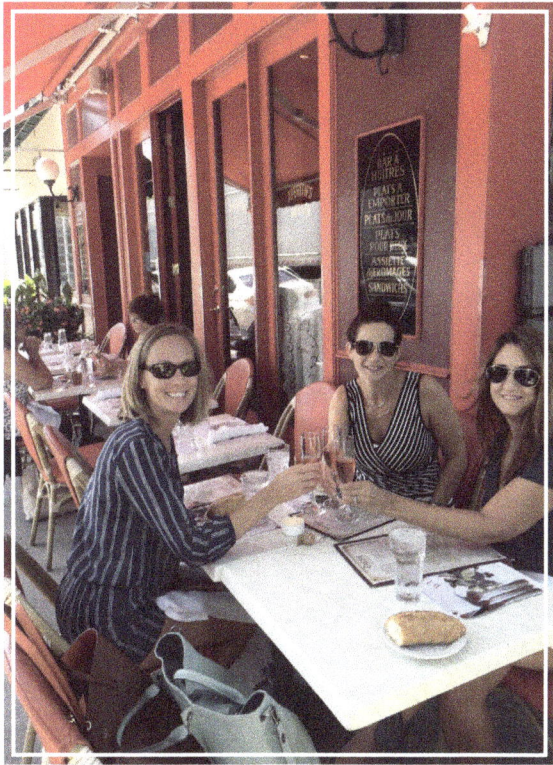
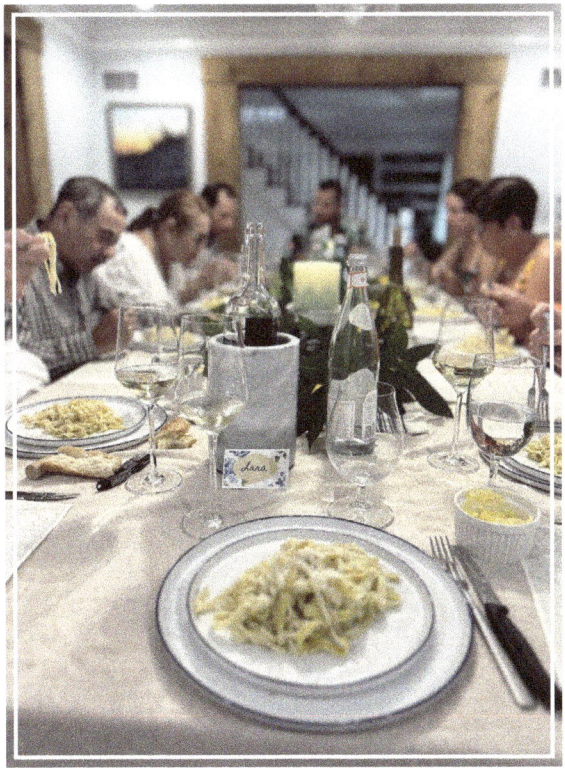
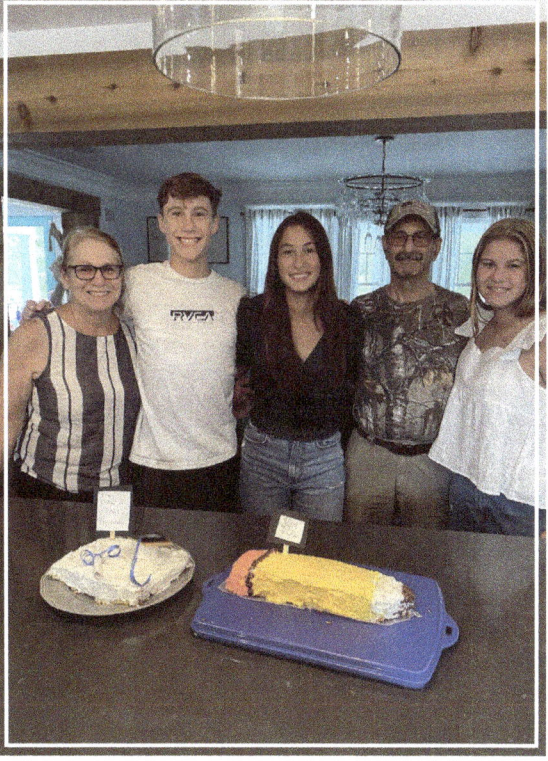

Quality time with family and friends often revolves around food

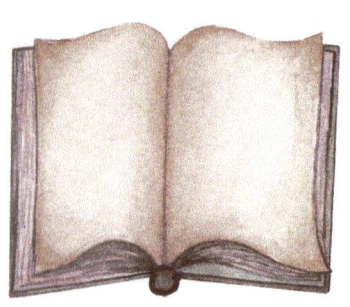

There are so many versions of Bibles out there:
the original Holy Bible, of course, but whatever you are into you can find:

The Squat Bible, by Aaron Horschig, Kevin Sonthana, and Travis Nef
The Juicing Bible, by Pat Crocker
The Chakra Bible, by Patricia Mercier
Cheese, Sex, Death, by Erica Kubick
The Hormone Balance Bible, by by Shawn A. Tassone

…….and believe it or not, the Christmas gift most cherished to my son,

The Snark Bible: A Reference Guide to Verbal Sparring, Comebacks, Irony, Insults, and So Much More by Lawrence Dorfman

May this book serve as your "Health Bible" and use it in good health. **Food is My Religion** intends to plant these seeds of nutrition, health and wellness for you to grow deep into roots of nutrition that branch out to support what nourishes us for lasting health habits for a life in full bloom.

There are many aspects of life that contribute to nutrition. It's not just what's on your plate, but the way you think, the way you feel, the way you pray, the way you move, the way you rest and sleep and the way you work. **Food is My Religion** provides an insight on how to pay attention to that all encompassing healthy lifestyle.

Whatever your religion and/or beliefs may be, there is an undeniable reason to have faith of some sort. Whatever you believe in spiritually, whether it is in a higher power, the universe or yourself. Having spirituality is beneficial for your overall health.

Read on for how and why we fuel our bodies with healthy ingredients, how you can believe in the power of food as medicine. I believe if you know the whys and why nots, you are more likely to make a change and stick with it. You will get some ideas on how to best set up your TEMPLE, your kitchen, where you will create healthy recipes and make lasting memories with yourself and loved ones.

You will also find some health centric rituals that may help create a calmer, more spiritual, best version of yourself; which in turn helps you show up for others. In part 2, I share recipes from my Temple, my kitchen. Plus, create some fantastic ways you can celebrate foods that nourish you.

> *"No disease that can be treated by diet should be treated with any other means."*
>
> –Maimonides

HOW WE EAT CAN BE JUST AS IMPORTANT AS WHAT WE EAT

The Sacred Ritual of Eating

Food is not just fuel; it is an experience, a communion between our senses and our bodies. In the hustle and bustle of modern life, we often overlook the importance of how we eat. Yet, the act of eating can be as significant as the food we put on our plates. To embrace food as a religion is to embrace not only its flavors but also the rituals that accompany it. This chapter invites you to slow down, engage your senses, and cultivate a mindful approach to nourishment.

Take a moment. Slow down. Inhale deeply, allowing the aromatic bouquet of your meal to awaken your senses. Do not rush through the experience; instead, immerse yourself in it. Imagine all this warm (or cool) goodness traveling down your digestive tract—a journey that goes beyond mere sustenance. It's important to recognize that within you lies a complex network, a vibrant community known as your microbiome.

What is the Microbiome?

Your microbiome is a vast ecosystem of trillions of microorganisms, primarily bacteria, residing in your intestines. These tiny allies play a crucial role in your health, influencing digestion, immune function, and even mental well-being. Picture this: the surface area of your intestines, when lined up, would cover the surface area of a tennis court! Within this expansive space, a joyful dance unfolds—a lively interplay of bacilli, each doing little jumps of joy, celebrating the nutrients you've just offered them. They thrive on variety, fiber, probiotics, and wholesome foods, transforming your meals into the energy that sustains you.

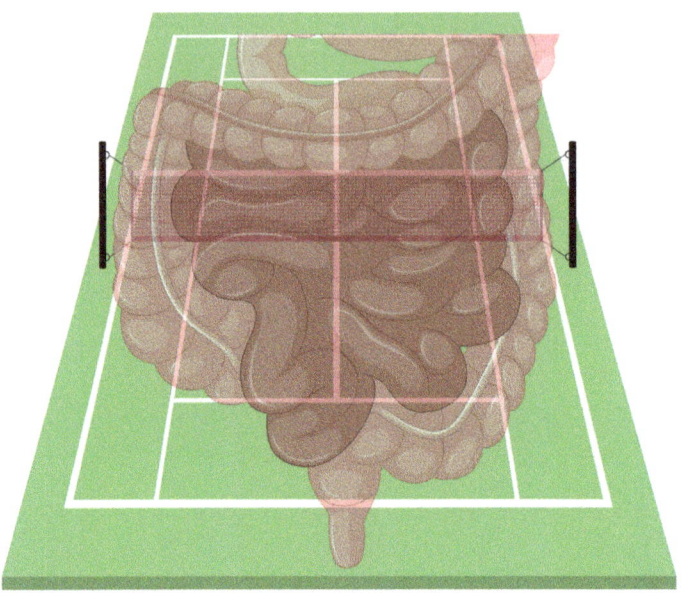

As you take the time to appreciate what's on your plate, understand that it is not just about the ingredients but also about the loving intention behind the meal. Our bodies are incredible machines capable of miraculous processes. They deserve care, respect, and dedication. This does not mean you have to adhere to strict rules of eating. Instead, you can find balance and joy in your meals.

In the following pages, I will guide you in constructing nutritious plates that reflect your unique needs and preferences. You will discover the elements that support your health and vitality and those sneaky ingredients that can thwart your good intentions. Every single person has different needs, likes and dislikes. This is a guide, which I find a great standard for all. By becoming knowledgeable about what to include and what to avoid, you can build a relationship with food that elevates your well-being.

Creating healthy rhythms is essential for your system to operate at its best. This means cultivating habits that support digestion, honoring your hunger cues, and embracing the mindfulness of each bite. Aim to establish routines that resonate with you, whether it's preparing a meal with loved ones, enjoying a quiet dinner, or savoring every flavor on your plate.

As we embark on this journey together, let us remember that food is more than sustenance; it is a ritual, a celebration of life itself. By honoring the how just as much as the what, we nourish not only our bodies but also our souls. So, let's dive deeper into the world of mindful eating—where the experience of food becomes a path to joy, health, and connection.

I believe in whole foods, healthy alternatives for treats, and occasional ways to let go.

THE YES LIST

Here's a list of whole foods to include in your lovely life (we will get to portion sizes next, don't worry):

While Amazon's Whole Foods, the store, certainly has the "Market" on the name, When I refer to "Whole Foods," I am referring to real foods that are natural, minimally processed, plants and animals sources of nutrition.

All Vegetables and All Fruit: Pure and simple if it comes from a plant, it's on the List! Aim for the rainbow every day and make a game of how many varieties of foods you can try to get in each and every day. Your body will thank you.

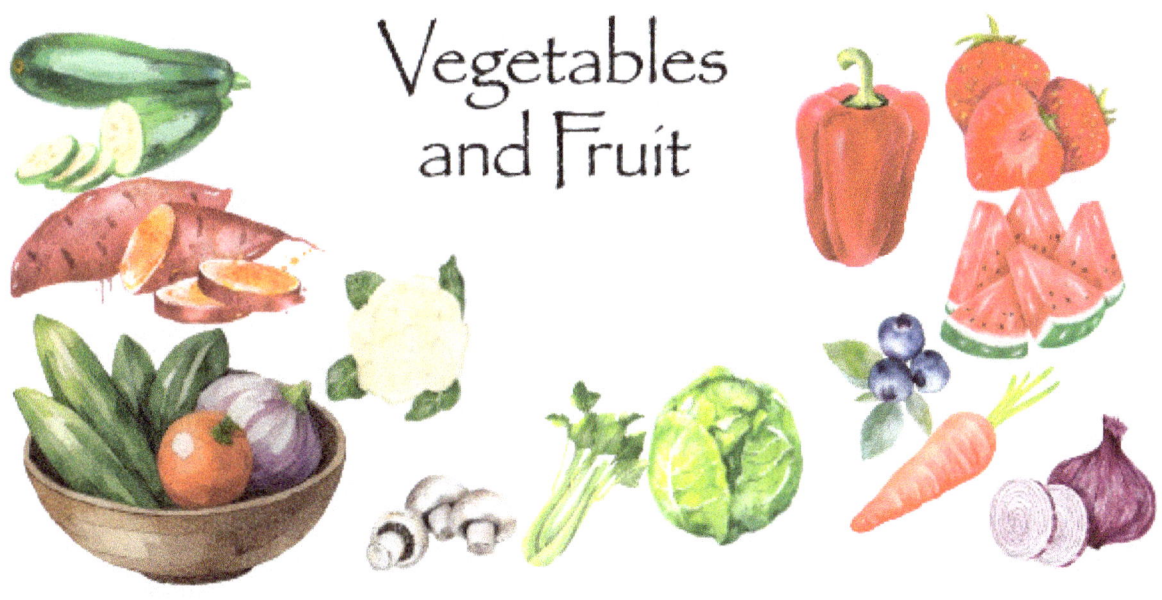

Protein: Beef (grass fed and organic are best), Chicken (free range and fed organic are best), Pork (no nitrates), Eggs (the best are from local free range, organic fed chickens), Fish and Shellfish (look for Wild Caught or sustainably raised, use this resource to see what's what https://www.seafoodwatch.org/), Lamb (Most lamb raised in the USA is sustainably grass fed) Organic Beans (Garbanzo, White Beans, Black Beans, Red Beans, etc.) lentils and legumes.

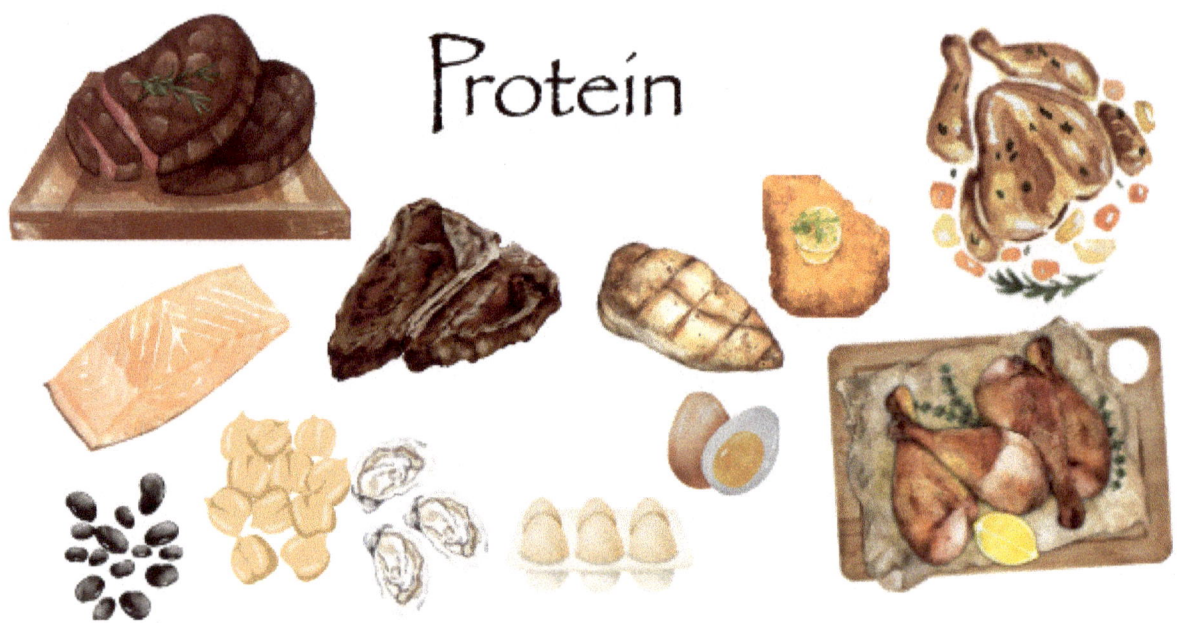

Bonus: Bone Broth - This nourishing nutrient powerhouse has healing effects. It's great for bone health, gut health and your immune system. There are many reputable brands out there, just remember to read ingredients, you are looking for pure bone broth. Sip on it any time you want, but especially between meals for a snack, or to stave off a virus if you start feeling under the weather. Make this a ritual by heating some broth, put it in your favorite mug as you would tea. Use your senses, smell how nourishing and feel it trickle down your digestive tract, knowing your microbes are welcoming it with healing broth.

Grains: Barley, Buckwheat, Coix, Farro, Millet, Oats, Quinoa, Rice

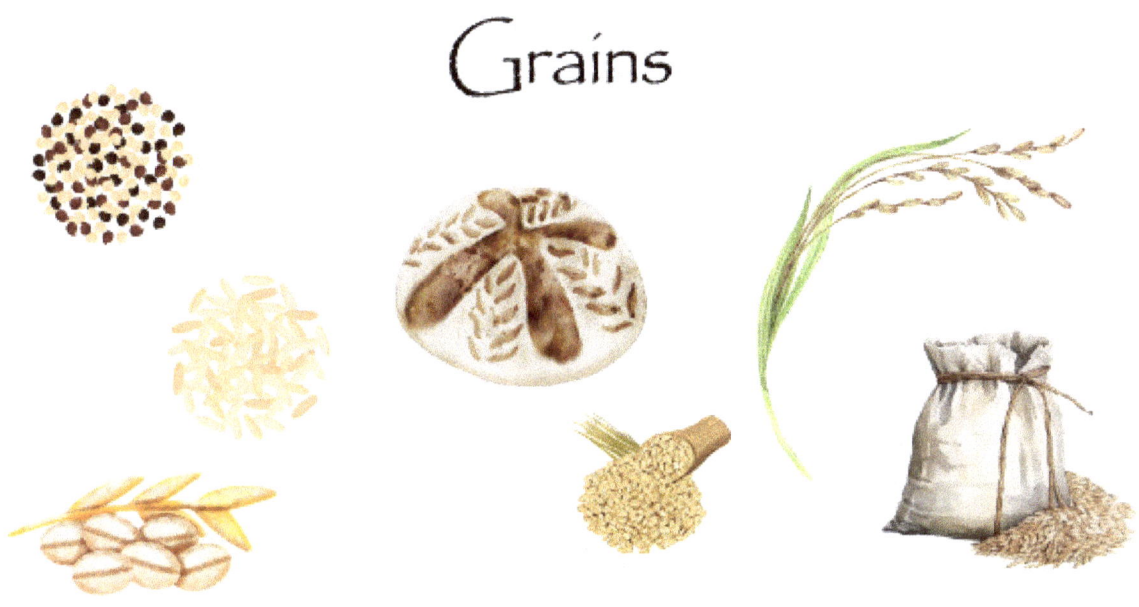

Bonus: Most of the time, opt for gluten free (gluten can be inflammatory, and we thrive with an anti-inflammatory diet), read on for more information on this.

When eating bread, choose something that has the fewest ingredients on the side of the package. Even better- opt to make your own experiment in your kitchen! We caught onto the sourdough craze during the COVID pandemic. Eternally grateful for our friend who shared her starter. You need what's called a starter, that is a mixture of flour and water that contains a good bacteria, wild yeast that is fermented, and used to leaven bread. Because sourdough goes through this fermentation process, it feeds your microbiome with probiotics and fiber, it has amazing healthy gut benefits and is easier to digest than standard bread.

Sourdough bread is not only delicious but also packed with health benefits that elevate it above many other types of bread. The unique fermentation process involves naturally occurring lactobacilli and wild yeasts, which not only impart a distinct tangy flavor but also enhance the bioavailability of nutrients. This means that minerals such as magnesium, iron, and zinc are more easily absorbed by the body. Additionally, the fermentation process lowers the bread's glycemic index, resulting in a slower release of glucose into the bloodstream, which can help regulate blood sugar levels. Sourdough is also easier to digest for many people compared to conventional bread, thanks to the breakdown of gluten during fermentation. Furthermore, its probiotic content can contribute to gut health, supporting a diverse microbiome. Including sourdough bread in your diet allows you to enjoy a flavorful experience while reaping these nutritional rewards.

A homemade sourdough bread is a fantastic way to end Passover and start eating leavened bread after only eating matzah for the duration of the jewish holiday passover. Sourdough starters can last years and years, generations even. No wonder it has caught on to the mainstream. Once the starter is established, you can share with friends and family, neighbors and strangers, it is just another way to connect, through food.

We named our sourdough starter "Jesus" because it was given to us around Easter time and it rises! My Mom's sourdough starter's name is "Moses." And because you need to feed it and discard some, it's great to share - some other disciples, it's fun to give it a name, of our sourdough starter, Jesus, are Mary, Merlin, Phoenix, St. Bernadette, Sunny and Freya.

Take a look at www.LandofNutrition.com/sourdough where I share more information about sourdough. Also Check out the book: *Artisan Bread in Five Minutes a Day* by Jeff Hertzberg and Zoë François and look up easy sourdough on Tik Tok or Instagram to get inspiration!

Did you know freezing bread can lower the glycemic index, creating a better situation for your health? Freezing bread is a simple yet effective technique that can play a significant role in managing glycemic index (GI) levels. When bread is frozen and then thawed, its starch structure undergoes a process called retrogradation, which alters how the carbohydrates are absorbed in the body. This reduces the glycemic response, meaning that the bread will cause a slower rise in blood sugar levels compared to freshly baked bread. By embracing the practice of freezing whole loaves or slices, you not only extend their shelf life but also enhance their nutritional profile. This small adjustment can make a substantial difference for those looking to regulate their blood sugar levels while still enjoying the comforting taste of bread—transforming a potential dietary challenge into a mindful choice, helping your body function in a better way.

Healthy Fats: Avocado, Avocado Oil, Olives, Extra Virgin Olive Oil, Grass Fed Butter, Coconut Oil and Ghee, Nuts & seeds - especially Almonds, Chia Seeds, Flax Seeds, Hemp Seeds, Pumpkin, Sesame, and Sunflower Seeds

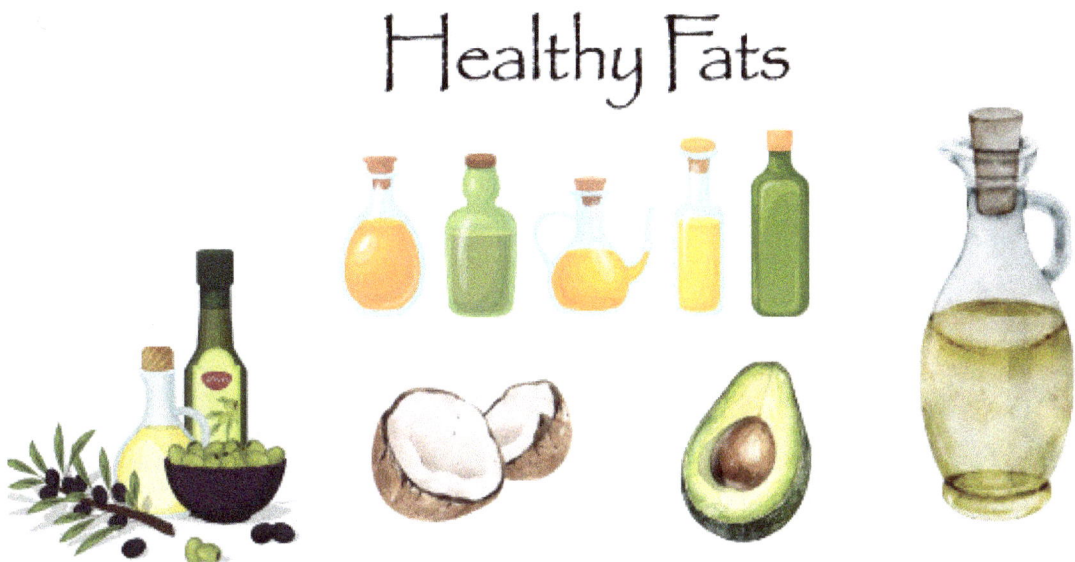

Herbs and Spices: Basil, Chili Powder, Chives, Cilantro, Cinnamon, Cumin, Garlic, Ginger, Mint, Oregano, Parsley, Pepper, Rosemary, Sea Salt, Tarragon, Thyme, Turmeric and so many more.

Dairy: Always opt for organic, grass fed Milk, Half & Half, Cream and Cheeses. Whole Milk Greek Yogurt, or Skyr Yogurt, if it is Organic, is a great choice. How about three cheers for Parmesan Cheese, *"Parmigiano Reggiano is naturally lactose free. The absence of lactose is a natural consequence of the traditional Parmigiano Reggiano manufacturing process. **Less than 0.01g / 100g galactose**."* Parmesan Reggiano also delivers 8g Protein per serving, making a great snack!

As with gluten, I have a caveat here. Some studies show that dairy is highly inflammatory, you can do the experiment on yourself by eliminating it for some time: 3 days to a month and slowly add it back to see how your body reacts.

Raw cheese is better for your gut. Look for organic cheese from grass fed cows, but don't eat raw cheeses if you are pregnant or breastfeeding.

Unbeknownst to you, the pre-shredded cheese you find at the grocery store is filled with additives to keep it from sticking together. Buy a block and shred it yourself.

If you are not lactose intolerant, Organic Greek Yogurt and Cheeses…enjoy it in moderation. Studies also show dairy can be inflammatory, in my opinion, a good chunk of parmesan cheese or an organic goat cheese can be much healthier than the "fake cheese" labeled vegan.

Hydration: Drink water, add cucumbers, strawberries, basil - get creative.

Club Soda or sparkling water that does not contain additional sugar or ambiguous ingredients ("natural flavoring" is a mystery, so avoid it).

Herbal Tea with some ice makes a great alternative to soda and sugary juices.

Bonus: Avoid store bought hydration drinks laden with artificial flavors and artificial colors.

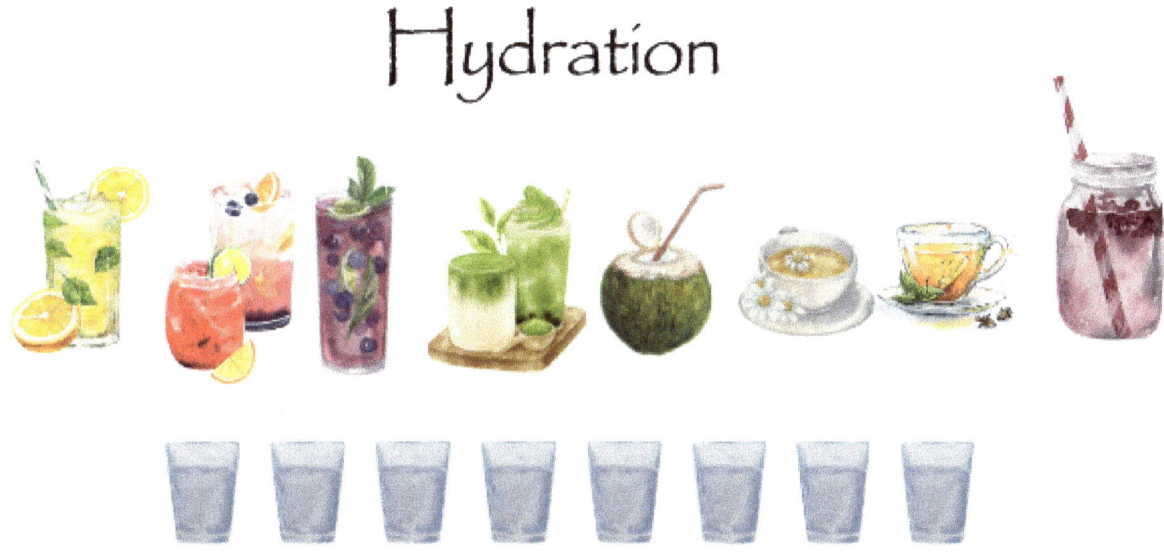

Worshiping food is okay, if it's done in a healthy way.

Believe in yourself to make the choices that are best for you. You do not have to stick to these principles 100% of the time, that could lead to a host of other problems. A good guide would be to choose the best options, 80%-90% of the time. This leaves room for your favorite treat once in a while. Special occasions are exactly that - an occasional treat is not going to wreck your overall health, obsessing about it can.

When you make your food choices a priority, your health will be a result. Knowing why these foods are beneficial can help you make the right choices.

When you want something sweet.....

Notice how Sugar is not on this list: Opt for a more natural sugar: maple syrup, banana, honey, dates. (We will get to this in the coming chapter: THE NAUGHTY LIST), but don't fret, there are so many great options, you will never miss it! Death by sugar may not be an overstatement—evidence is mounting that sugar is THE MAJOR FACTOR causing obesity and chronic disease.

Choosing a diverse selection of natural, unprocessed, whole foods helps your body to benefit from the different nutrients each group and within each group has to offer.

Think of vegetables and fruits in terms of protecting you with their vitamins, minerals, enzymes, and beneficial phytonutrients, polyphenols, all which moderate negative metabolic effects of too much processed foods: high blood pressure, high blood sugar, insulin resistance, chronic illnesses, heart disease.

LAND OF NUTRITION SHIELD

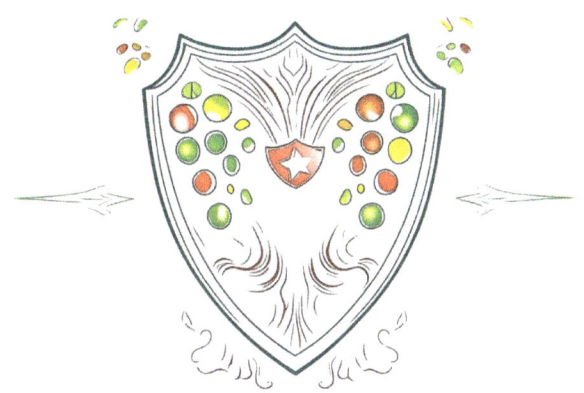

What you do now in terms of nutrition, how you take care of yourself now, what you put on your plate now will affect you in 5,10-20 years from now. Nutrition can be used as a preventative measure for chronic illness that is affecting 1 in 3 Americans.

Food can heal or food can harm
~ let food be your daily treatment.

Organic and regenerative farming is one way to help negate the effects - a priority in this day and age, where most food for most people comes from a processing plant. Let's end this and get out in our own gardens, you don't need much space, you can plant herbs, and my favorite, kale, just about anywhere that gets some sunlight and water. In the next chapter we will dive into the why's and why nots and best sources of each category.

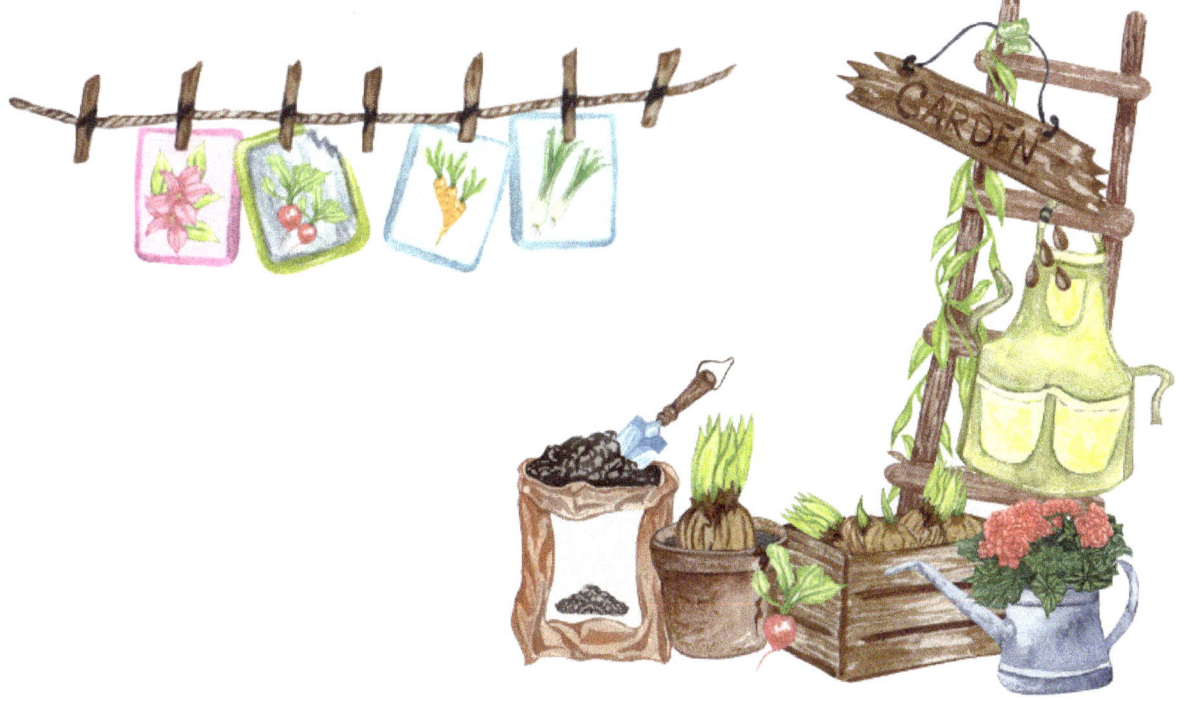

FOOD IS MY RELIGION
I WORSHIP FOOD AND THE NOURISHMENT WE GET FROM IT

THE WHY's BEHIND WHOLE FOODS:

Vegetables, Fruit, Protein, Healthy Fats, Grains, Herbs, Spices and Hydration

YES LIST:

VEGETABLES and FRUIT

Vegetables and Fruits are an important part of your plate due to the endless health benefits. Phytochemicals, polyphenols and antioxidants in vegetables and fruit help protect against many chronic diseases. **Aim to fill half of your plate with** vegetables.

Here are some of the key reasons why fruits and vegetables, a diet rich in fiber provided by plants, are good for you:

- ✓ Cancer and Heart Disease Prevention
- ✓ Decrease the risk of cardiovascular disease
- ✓ Inhibit the growth and development of cancerous cells
- ✓ Regulate blood pressure levels by keeping blood vessels healthy and flexible and promote good circulation
- ✓ Reduce chronic inflammation which leads to chronic illness and heart disease
- ✓ Gain control of blood sugar by slowing the conversion of carbohydrates into simple sugars after meals, lowering the risk of type 2 diabetes
- ✓ Fiber for Gut Health: Fruits and vegetables are excellent sources of fiber, which supports the immune system and gut microbiome. Fiber also helps prevent constipation and reduces the risk of diverticulosis.

- ✓ Eye Health: Vitamins, minerals and antioxidants like lutein in colorful fruits and veggies help prevent age-related eye diseases and promote healthy vision. Have you ever seen a bunny wearing glasses?
- ✓ Strong Bones: Vitamins C, K and A, along with minerals like magnesium and potassium found in produce, are important for building bone density and preventing osteoporosis.
- ✓ Immune Boosting: High levels of vitamins C and A in many fruits and vegetables strengthen the immune system.
- ✓ Weight Management: Fruits and veggies are low in calories but high in volume, helping you feel full and satisfied to aid in weight control.
- ✓ There's more - by filling half of your plate at each meal with veggies and fruit you can stave away Illness with these amazing antioxidant effects
- ✓ Reduce inflammation in the body, protect against oxidative stress, slow cellular aging
- ✓ Protect against neurodegenerative diseases by reducing oxidative stress in the brain, potentially lowering the risk of conditions like Alzheimer's and Parkinson's disease
- ✓ Enhance your microbiome, your beneficial gut bacteria and Inhibit the growth of potentially harmful bacteria
- ✓ Glowing Skin, defend against oxidative stress from sun exposure and pollution, slowing external skin aging and reducing wrinkles, Plants are a great source for detoxifying free radicals (Harmful chemicals in our skincare, laundry and haircare products, smog, cigarette smoke, nicotine vape)

Think of it like this:

Apples improve digestion with fiber, support heart health, and help balance blood sugar.
Avocados provide healthy fats, support hormone balance, and nourish the brain.
Beets support liver health, improve blood flow, and boost stamina with natural nitrates.
Blueberries fight inflammation, sharpen memory, and help keep blood sugar stable.
Broccoli detoxifies the body, balances hormones, and contains compounds linked to cancer prevention.
Carrots are rich in beta-carotene, which promotes eye health, glowing skin, and a stronger immune system.
Cilantro promotes detoxification and boosts immunity.
Cucumbers hydrate, cool the body, support skin health, aid in weight loss, and promote eye health.
Garlic strengthens immunity, reduces blood pressure, and fights harmful bacteria and viruses.
Kale is nutrient-dense with vitamins A, C, and K, building strong bones and promoting detoxification.
Mushrooms boost vitamin D, support gut health, and enhance immune defense.
Onions are a superfood reducing risks of chronic illness and cancer.
Pineapple aids digestion with natural enzymes, fights inflammation, and strengthens joints.
Purple Cabbage is loaded with antioxidants, supports detoxification, and helps reduce inflammation.
Red Bell Peppers deliver more vitamin C than oranges, strengthening immunity and promoting collagen for youthful skin.
Spinach is packed with iron, folate, and antioxidants that strengthen bones, aid energy, and support brain health.
Strawberries protect heart health, support glowing skin, and help regulate blood sugar.
Tomatoes are full of lycopene, a powerful antioxidant that protects the heart and lowers cancer risk.

You get the gist!
The key here is to "eat the rainbow" by consuming a variety of colorful fruits and vegetables to get a wide range of beneficial nutrients.

Let's play a game by listing all the different varieties you can get in for the week!

Red

Red foods are packed with lycopene and anthocyanins, powerful antioxidants that help protect against heart disease and certain cancers. They also provide vitamins like C and A, support healthy skin, boost immunity, and promote good circulation.

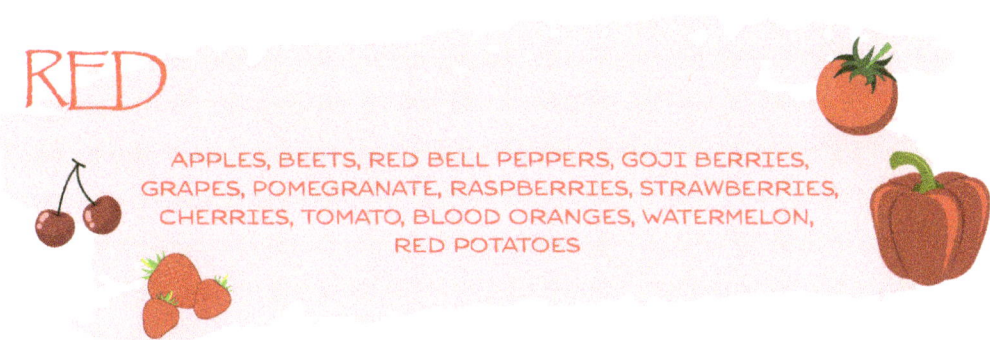

Orange / Yellow

Orange and yellow foods are rich in beta-carotene, which boosts vision, immunity, and skin health. They also provide antioxidants, vitamin C, fiber, and potassium, supporting heart health and digestion.

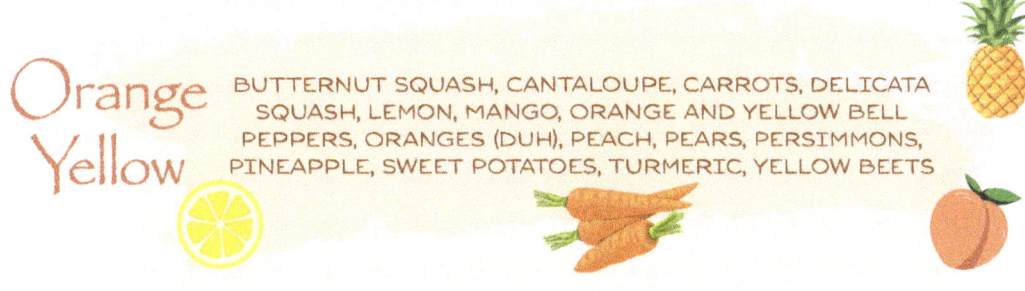

Greens are extra special

Greens are packed with fiber, folate, calcium, magnesium, potassium, iron, and a wealth of vitamins. They support circulation, detoxification, immunity, heart health, digestion, liver function, and cell regeneration.

Green: ASPARAGUS, BOK CHOY, BROCCOLI, BRUSSEL SPROUTS, CABBAGE, CELERY, CILANTRO, CUCUMBERS, DULSE SEAWEED, GRAPES, GREEN BEANS, KALE, KIWI, LETTUCE OF ALL KINDS, MINT, PARSLEY, SAGE, SCALLIONS, SNAP AND SWEET PEAS, ZUCCHINI

Blue / Purple / Black

Blue and purple fruits and veggies get their color from anthocyanins, powerful antioxidants that support heart and brain health, reduce inflammation, and may lower cancer risk. They're also rich in fiber and vitamins, making them a tasty and healthy addition to any meal.

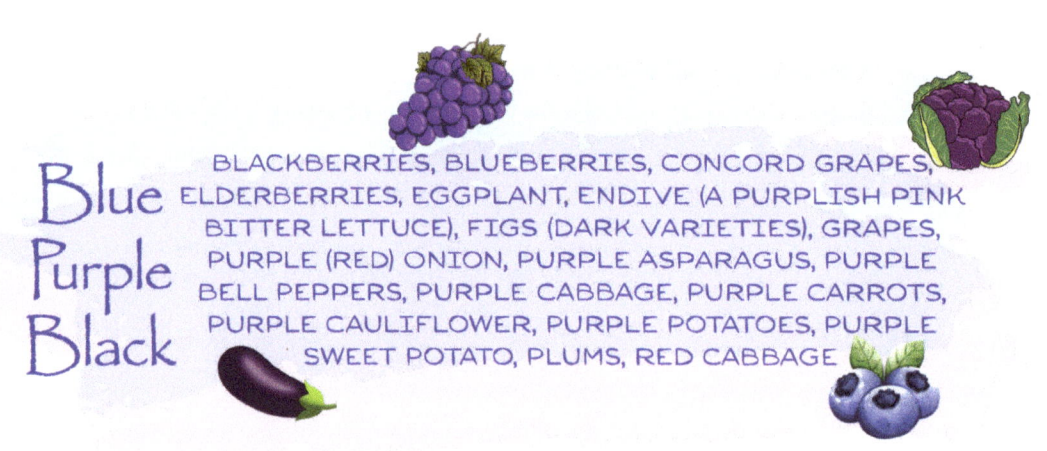

Blue Purple Black: BLACKBERRIES, BLUEBERRIES, CONCORD GRAPES, ELDERBERRIES, EGGPLANT, ENDIVE (A PURPLISH PINK BITTER LETTUCE), FIGS (DARK VARIETIES), GRAPES, PURPLE (RED) ONION, PURPLE ASPARAGUS, PURPLE BELL PEPPERS, PURPLE CABBAGE, PURPLE CARROTS, PURPLE CAULIFLOWER, PURPLE POTATOES, PURPLE SWEET POTATO, PLUMS, RED CABBAGE

White

White fruits and vegetables are rich in phytonutrients like allicin and flavonoids that support heart health, reduce inflammation, and boost the immune system. They often contain fiber, potassium, and vitamins C and B6, which help with digestion, blood pressure regulation, and overall wellness. Adding white produce brings gentle but powerful health benefits to your diet.

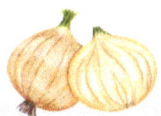
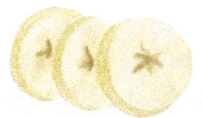

White: BANANAS, BAMBOO SHOOTS, CAULIFLOWER, COCONUT, DAIKON RADISH, DATES, FENNEL, GARLIC, HEARTS OF PALM, JICAMA, KOHLRABI (WHITE VARIETY), LYCHEE, MUSHROOMS, NAPA CABBAGE, ONION, PARSNIPS, PEARS (ASIAN OR BARTLETT), POTATOES, SHALLOTS, TURNIPS, WHITE ASPARAGUS, WHITE CORN, WHITE EGGPLANT, WHITE MUSHROOMS, WHITE NECTARINES, WHITE PEACHES

Try dried fruit and veggies like Kale Chips and Dried Tart Cherries (Just watch the ingredients for no added sugar or that anything from the naughty list doesn't wreck your good intentions).

How many varieties did you get in a day?

In a week? This Month?

Keep your list here:

PROTEIN

Why you should include it:

Protein is an essential macronutrient that plays a critical role in the body.
Here are several reasons why protein is important for your diet.

- ✓ Muscle Growth: Consuming adequate protein helps stimulate muscle protein synthesis, which is necessary for muscle growth and strength, especially important for just about everyone aging. In her book *Forever Strong*, Dr. Gabrielle Lyon emphasizes that our muscular system is key to longevity, underscoring the vital role of protein.
- ✓ Building and Repairing Tissues: Protein is vital for the growth, repair, and maintenance of body tissues, including muscles, skin, organs, and hair.
- ✓ Hormone Production: Many hormones including glucagon, insulin, thyroid, estrogen, testosterone, progesterone, cortisol, are made up of proteins. These hormones regulate various bodily functions, including metabolism, growth, and mood.
- ✓ Enzyme Function: Proteins act as enzymes that facilitate biochemical reactions in the body, essential for processes such as digestion and metabolism.
- ✓ Immune Function: Antibodies, which are proteins, play a crucial role in the immune system by identifying and neutralizing pathogens like bacteria and viruses.
- ✓ Weight Management: Protein-rich foods can help promote satiety, which can reduce overall calorie intake and assist in weight management by keeping you feeling fuller for longer.
- ✓ Healthy Hair, Skin, and Nails: Proteins are significant components of hair, skin, and nails, contributing to their strength and appearance.
- ✓ Blood Sugar Regulation: Including protein in meals can help stabilize blood sugar levels by slowing digestion and absorption of carbohydrates, which can prevent spikes and crashes in blood sugar.
- ✓ Energy Source: While carbohydrates and fats are the primary sources of energy, proteins can also be used for energy when necessary, especially during prolonged fasting or intense exercise.
- ✓ Supports Healthy Aging: Adequate protein intake can help reduce muscle loss associated with aging (sarcopenia) and support overall health and mobility in older adults.
- ✓ To meet your protein needs, it's important to include a variety of protein sources in your diet, such as meat, fish, dairy, legumes, nuts, seeds, and whole grains.

How to get enough protein:

Each of 3 meals aim for 30 grams of protein, probably a lot more than you think.
What that looks like (note how much more you would need of the plant based protein):

- *6oz Grass Fed Steak or Grass Fed Ground Beef Burger*
- *About 10 Large Shrimp*
- *5 Large Organic Free Range Eggs*
- *A large palm size piece of free range chicken breast, Turkey, Pork, wild caught Salmon or Cod*
- *1 Cup of Organic Cottage Cheese or 1 1/2 Cup Organic Greek Yogurt*
- *1 Cup Organic Tempeh*
- *2 Cups of Black Beans (this can be a lot of beans to eat at once, so add in moderation to enhance protein servings)*

Bone broth offers several health benefits, making it a popular addition to many diets. Here are some key benefits:

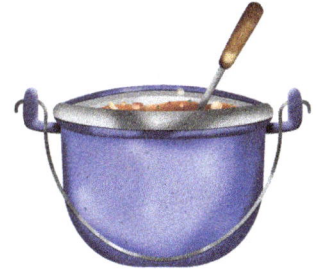

- ✓ Rich in Nutrients: Bone broth is packed with vitamins and minerals, such as calcium, magnesium, phosphorus, and vitamins A and K, which are essential for bone health.
- ✓ Supports Joint Health: The collagen and gelatin in bone broth can help improve joint health by providing nutrients that support cartilage and reduce inflammation.
- ✓ Improves Gut Health: Bone broth contains amino acids like glutamine, which may help support a healthy gut lining and promote digestive health.
- ✓ Boosts Immune System: The nutrients in bone broth can help strengthen the immune system, potentially reducing the risk of illness.
- ✓ Promotes Healthy Skin: The collagen found in bone broth can enhance skin elasticity and hydration, contributing to a youthful appearance.
- ✓ Aids in Hydration: Bone broth can contribute to hydration, especially during hot weather or after a workout, due to its mineral content and fluids.
- ✓ May Help with Weight Management: Bone broth is low in calories and can be filling, which might help control appetite and support weight loss efforts.
- ✓ Improves Sleep and Mood: The glycine found in bone broth may promote better sleep and improved mood by supporting neurotransmitter function.

Space to jot down your favorite protein:

HEALTHY FATS

Healthy fats are an essential part of a balanced diet and offer a range of health benefits.

A serving about the size of your thumb is great at each meal.
Incorporating monounsaturated, healthy fats from sources like avocados, nuts, seeds, olive oil, and fatty fish into your diet can provide benefits while supporting overall health. It's important to note these healthier options while limiting saturated and trans fats.

- ✓ Heart Health: Healthy fats, such as monounsaturated and polyunsaturated fats, can help lower bad cholesterol (LDL) levels while raising good cholesterol (HDL) levels, reducing the risk of heart disease and stroke
- ✓ Inflammation Reduction: Omega-3 fatty acids, which are found in fatty fish, walnuts, and flaxseeds, have anti-inflammatory properties that can help reduce inflammation in the body, promoting better overall health.
- ✓ Brain Function: Healthy fats are crucial for brain health. The brain is made up of around 60% fat, and adequate fat intake supports cognitive function, memory, and mood regulation.
- ✓ Nutrient Absorption: Certain vitamins (A, D, E, and K) are fat-soluble, meaning they require dietary fat for proper absorption. Consuming healthy fats can help ensure that your body efficiently absorbs these essential nutrients.
- ✓ Satiation and Weight Management: Healthy fats can help you feel full and satisfied, reducing cravings for unhealthy snacks and promoting better portion control.
- ✓ Hormonal Balance: Fats are necessary for the production of hormones, including sex hormones and hormones that help regulate metabolism. Healthy fats support overall hormonal balance.
- ✓ Healthy Skin and Hair: Fats contribute to maintaining healthy skin and hair by supporting the skin barrier and providing moisture. Omega-3 fatty acids, in particular, can help with skin conditions like dryness and inflammation.
- ✓ Energy Source: Fats serve as a concentrated source of energy, providing more than double the calories per gram than carbohydrates or proteins. This can be beneficial for sustained energy during prolonged physical activities.
- ✓ Support Cellular Function: Fats are a key component of cell membranes, helping to maintain their integrity and fluidity, which is essential for proper cell function.
- ✓ Flavor and Culinary Enjoyment: Healthy fats, such as those found in avocados, nuts, and olive oil, enhance the flavor of foods, making meals more enjoyable and satisfying.

Extra Virgin Olive Oil "EVOO" is best in salad dressings and low heat points sautéing veggies. Olive Oil has a high smoke point - between 365-420° - so you don't want to heat it up too much, the beneficial compounds start to deteriorate and cause adverse health effects. Anything over 380° F (193° C) could start to create harmful free radicals, the very thing we are looking to avoid.

EVOO has those polyphenols, vitamins E and helps to absorb the fat-soluble vitamins (A, D, E, & K). Look for a Dark Glass bottle and make sure it's extra-virgin, cold or expeller-pressed with a harvest date, rather than expiration date.

For higher heat use Avocado Oil, Coconut oil, Ghee, Coconut oil, or butter.
Other great Healthy Fats to include are avocado, nuts and seeds, ground flax seed, unsweetened dried coconut flakes makes a great snack and addition to your trail mix.

Nutty Ideas for healthy fats:

Almonds (my grandfather would eat a handful a day for health and he lived a LONG fruitful life), Brazil Nuts (these are great for your thyroid, as they contain selenium), Cashews, Pine Nuts, Walnuts, Pistachios, hazelnuts are also good for protein, magnesium, and iron.

Pumpkin Seeds - Find minerals like magnesium, iron, and zinc. One ounce of pumpkin seeds can provide about a third of your recommended daily magnesium intake!
Add them to salads: Try sunflower seeds, flax seeds, sesame seeds, hemp seeds.

Space to jot down your favorite healthy fats:

GRAINS

While whole grains have existed since the beginning of civilization, today's growing standards are sub par. Hold high grain standards by opting for whole grains, keeping them organic and gluten free. Studies show gluten can be inflammatory, so here is my reminder to choose organic and gluten free options when you can.

The body uses grains slowly, they provide sustained energy, and a source of enzymes, iron, and fiber.

- ✓ Nutrient-Rich: Whole grains are rich in essential nutrients, including vitamins (such as B vitamins), minerals (like iron and magnesium), and antioxidants. These nutrients are crucial for various bodily functions.
- ✓ High in Fiber: Whole grains are an excellent source of dietary fiber, which helps improve digestion, promotes regular bowel movements, and can prevent constipation. Fiber also plays a role in maintaining a healthy gut microbiome.
- ✓ Heart Health: Consuming whole grains is associated with a reduced risk of heart disease. The fiber, antioxidants, and healthy fats found in whole grains can help lower cholesterol levels and improve heart health.
- ✓ Weight Management: High fiber content in whole grains promotes satiety, helping you feel full longer. This can assist with weight management by reducing overall calorie intake and preventing overeating.
- ✓ Blood Sugar Control: Whole grains have a lower glycemic index compared to refined grains, meaning they cause a slower, steadier rise in blood sugar levels. This can benefit individuals with diabetes or insulin resistance by helping to maintain stable blood sugar levels.
- ✓ Reduced Risk of Chronic Diseases: Diets rich in whole grains have been linked to a lower risk of various chronic diseases, including type 2 diabetes, certain cancers, and obesity.
- ✓ Improved Digestive Health: The fiber in whole grains supports healthy digestion and may help prevent gastrointestinal issues, such as diverticulitis, by promoting regular bowel movements.
- ✓ Energy Source: Grains provide complex carbohydrates, which are an important source of energy for the body, especially for those who are physically active.
- ✓ Versatility: Healthy grains can be incorporated into a wide variety of dishes, making it easy to add them to your diet. Options include brown rice, quinoa, oats, whole wheat bread, and barley.
- ✓ Sustainable Foods: Many whole grains have a lower environmental impact compared to highly processed foods. Choosing whole grains can be a part of a sustainable and health-conscious lifestyle.

- *Try some favorites: Brown Rice, Wild Rice, Buckwheat, Oats, Quinoa, Farro.*
- *One Cup of uncooked grains can vary anywhere from 2-4 servings.*
- *Take the time to experiment here, like with any food, and see how you feel. What works for one person may be different from another, even in your own household.*

Space to jot down your favorite grains:

You are your best advocate.

HYDRATION

Drink Water Throughout the day- aim for 64-80oz, about 8 cups or half of your body weight in ounces. So if you weigh 160lbs, you can aim for 80oz of water.

Staying hydrated is crucial for overall health and well-being. Here are the main reasons why hydration is important:

- ✓ Hydration significantly affects brain function. Dehydration can lead to difficulties in concentration, increased feelings of anxiety, and impaired memory. Studies show that even slight fluid loss can negatively impact mood and cognitive abilities.
- ✓ Prevents Headaches: Dehydration is a common trigger for headaches and migraines. Drinking sufficient water can alleviate headache symptoms and reduce their frequency.
- ✓ Aids Digestion: Water is vital for digestive health. It helps prevent constipation by facilitating bowel movements and is essential for the proper functioning of the digestive system.
- ✓ Regulates Body Temperature: Water plays a crucial role in thermoregulation. It helps maintain body temperature through sweating and respiration, which is particularly important in hot conditions or during intense physical activity.
- ✓ Supports Physical Performance, Adequate hydration is essential for optimal physical performance. Even mild dehydration can impair strength, endurance, and overall athletic performance, making exercise feel more challenging and increasing fatigue levels.
- ✓ Promotes Heart Health: Staying hydrated helps the heart pump blood more efficiently, reducing the workload on the heart. Proper hydration supports cardiovascular health by maintaining blood volume and circulation.
- ✓ Facilitates Nutrient Transport - Water is necessary for transporting nutrients and oxygen to cells, as well as removing waste products from the body. It ensures that essential bodily functions operate smoothly.
- ✓ Maintains Joint Health: Lubricate your joints, which is vital for reducing friction during movement and preventing joint pain or discomfort.

Hopefully this will prompt you to keep sipping throughout your day.

Our active bodies need electrolytes, which we lose when we sweat!

What are Electrolytes? Sodium, Calcium, Magnesium, Potassium, Chloride, Phosphorus

Sodium (Na): Salt (Sea Salt, Celtic Salt or Himalayan - NOT TABLE SALT), pickles, olives, whole grain pretzels or crackers

Calcium (Ca): Leafy Greens, Tahini, figs, Dairy (though inflammatory)

Magnesium (Mg): Spinach, Quinoa, Beans and Lentils, Nuts, Seeds

Potassium (K): Bananas, Squash, Broccoli, Potatoes, Orange

Chloride (Ci): Tomatoes, Leafy Greens, Olives, Seaweed, Salt

Phosphorus (P): Whole Wheat (Organic), cheese, PB, Corn, Broccoli, Chicken, Garlic, Nuts

What are NOT Electrolytes? Artificial Colors and Flavors. Many of the dyes and chemicals have been linked to cancer in lab animals, hyperactivity, ADHD, ADD, certain chronic illnesses and disease. Some studies show that brand name sports drinks are contributing to the obesity epidemic in children.

You can make your own homemade electrolyte drink:

- ✓ Enhance your water by adding a pinch of sea salt, and a squeeze of lemon
- ✓ For more complete electrolyte replenishment, include some potassium (like juice from a fresh squeezed orange) and a small amount of honey
- ✓ Make a juice by blending water, lemon, celery, apple, and celtic salt
- ✓ Mash Strawberry, lime juice with Pink Himalayan salt
- ✓ Coconut Water is a great choice
- ✓ Add chia seeds to your water for protein and a fun bubble drink!
- ✓ Or make a Smoothie: Frozen Banana, Almond Butter, Spinach or Kale leaves, Almond Milk, some fresh grated ginger

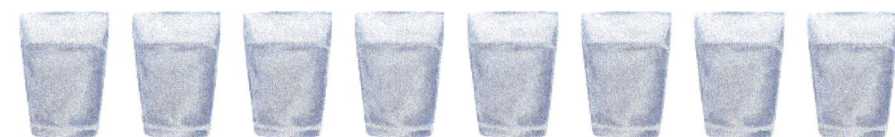

Space to jot down your favorite hydration hacks and keep track of your hydration:

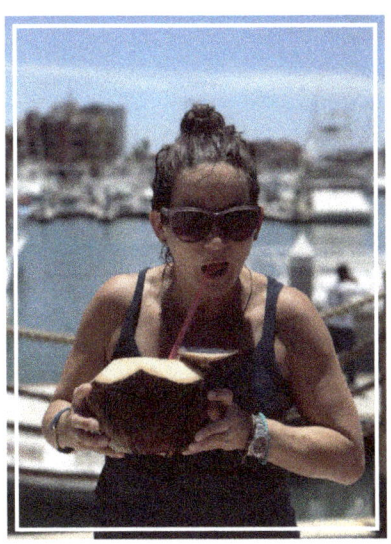 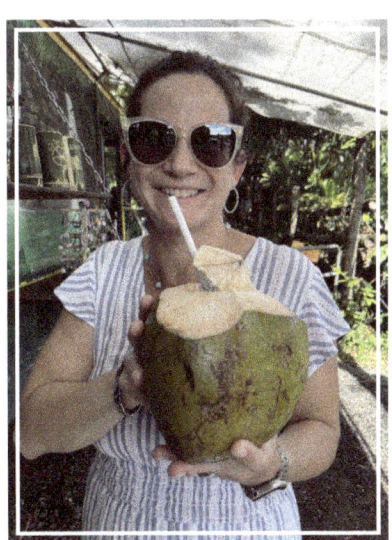 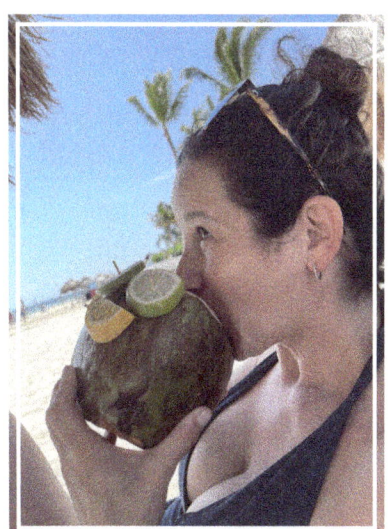

I love coconut water and traveling!

> *"If it came from a plant, eat it;*
> *if it was made in a plant, don't."*
>
> *~ Michael Pollan*

When it's important to use organic, and when you don't have to:
If you take a look at a fruit or vegetable's skin, you can make a determination based on how thick or thin the plant's skin is. For example, a strawberry has a very thin skin, herbicides and pesticides penetrate easily, so it's good to buy organic. A cantaloupe's outer layer is thick, the pesticides have a harder time seeping into the skin, so it's okay to buy conventionally grown. I recommend always washing fruits and veggies to deter contamination from farm workers or grocery store hands. I wash avocados and lemons with dish soap and my hand, rinsing completely to get rid of any residue. For leafy greens or berries soak with a vegetable wash made from baking soda or vinegar.

The Environmental Working Group, EWG, is a health and wellness advocacy group, a great resource for agriculture and household product safety. They do the dirty work for us by providing an annual list, the "Dirty Dozen," vegetables and fruits which have the most concentrations of pesticides and herbicides, it is recommended to buy organically grown.

The "Clean 15" are produce that you can feel safe buying conventionally grown vegetables and fruits, as they are less likely to find toxins. I highly recommend you visit for yourself, give a small donation and get the cute little card you can print out and keep in your wallet.

When you start to look at your produce from this angle, it helps to save money and time while selecting the most nutrient dense foods, after all, that is the goal here.

Foods with Highest Pesticides, choose organic here:

"Dirty Dozen" Always buy Organic,
Hint: **the grocery number will have a "9" in front:**

- ✓ Strawberries, I'll add: all berries
- ✓ Spinach, Kale, I say: all leafy greens
- ✓ Nectarines, Peaches, Apples, Pears
- ✓ Grapes, Cherries
- ✓ Celery
- ✓ Hot Peppers
- ✓ Tomatoes, Potatoes

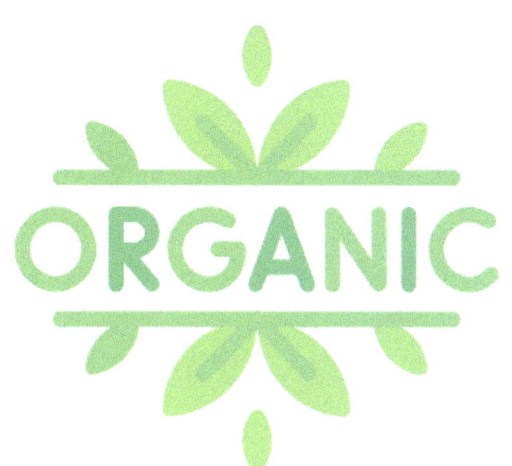

"Clean Fifteen" - Okay to buy Conventionally Grown

- ✓ Avocados
- ✓ Sweet Corn, Peas
- ✓ Pineapples, Papaya
- ✓ Onions, Cabbage
- ✓ Eggplants
- ✓ Asparagus
- ✓ Kiwi
- ✓ Cauliflower, Broccoli
- ✓ Cantaloupe, Honey Melons
- ✓ Mushrooms
- ✓ Bananas

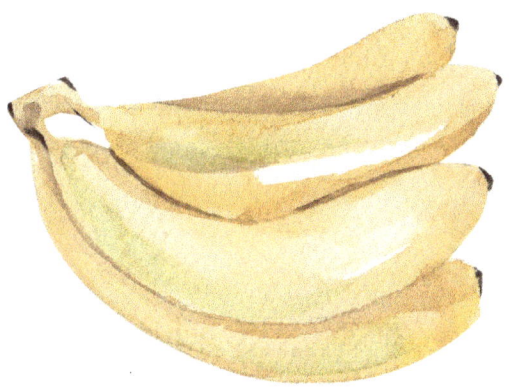

There is no doubt - more and more research is coming out to support claims that chronic illness can be controlled or reversed. Obliterate Diabetes, Alzheimers, Thyroid disease with good quality food. Eliminate processed foods and integrate whole foods to live a quality life.

It's no coincidence that with the rise in popularity of highly processed vegetable oils (such as soybean, canola, corn, and peanut), heart conditions have skyrocketed. These oils are cheap! So you will most likely find them hiding or in plain sight in restaurants, school lunches, college campuses, amusement parks, sports arenas, and more. Cooking at home gives you the best result for eating as healthy as possible. Remember, an occasional night out will not wreck your delicate and yet hardy system, just be aware of where your meals are coming from. There are many restaurants and food delivery services that, in fact, have healthier options.

> I believe in top quality food, gathering food from local sources, and eating seasonally as much as possible.

There's something about knowing the farmers and growers that brings us back to our roots. I also believe in growing some of your own. Microbes in soil can improve our health, love digging in the dirt? Studies show that kids that play in the yard, literally dig in the dirt, can have better immune systems, so why not make friends with the earth worms and take into consideration your own vegetable patch? You don't need acres to farm, just a small pot with herbs is a great start!

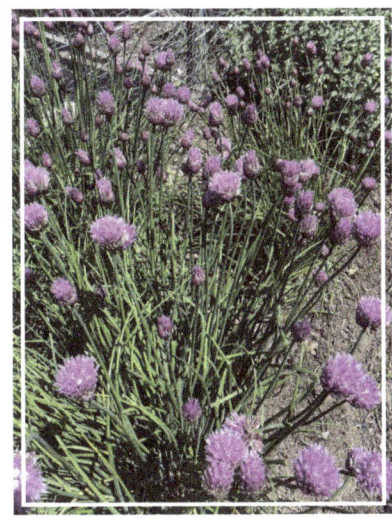
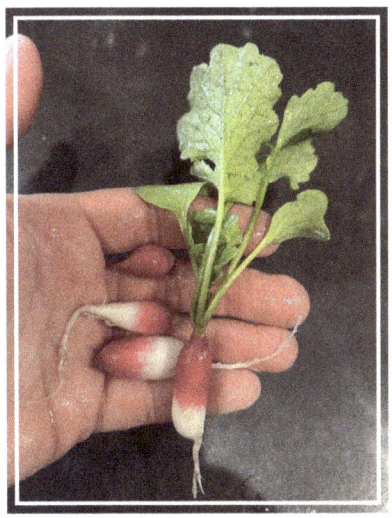
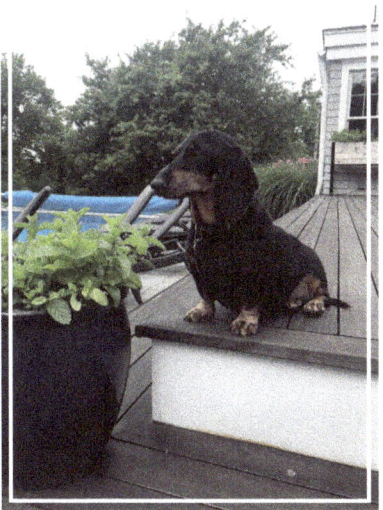
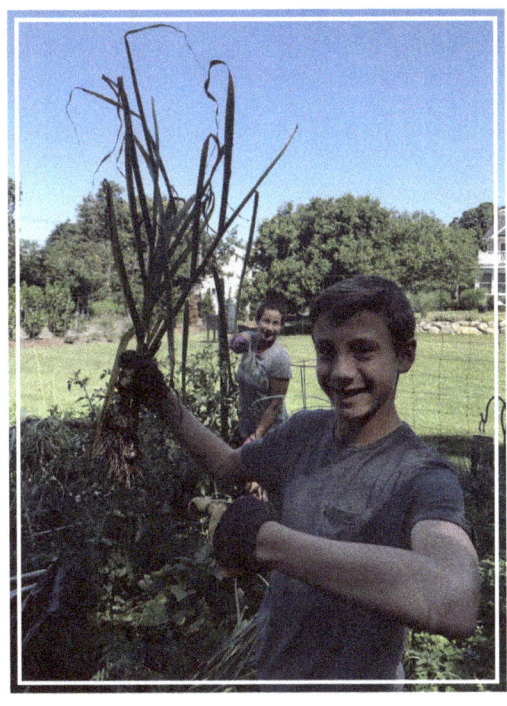
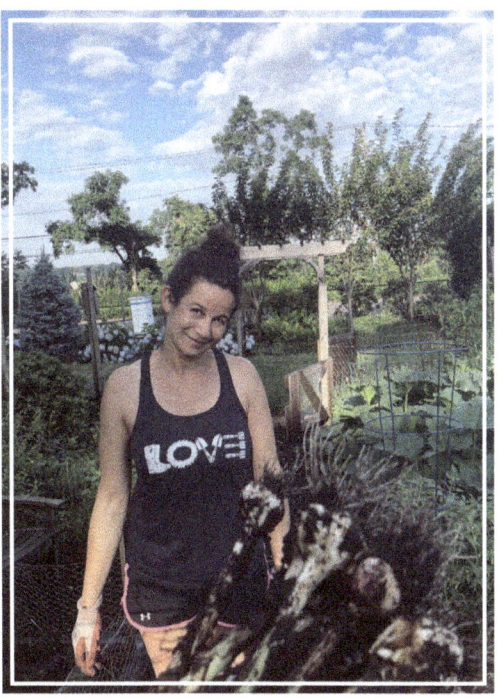

You will feel better, stave off disease and be happier when you cosume more fresh veggies.

With Community Supported Agriculture (CSA) or local Farmers Markets, you can get a variety of veggies and fruits grown seasonally, like mother nature intended. CSAs are gaining more and more local popularity, wherever you may live, since consumers are caring more about where their food comes from. This is a great way for individuals and families to reap the benefits of local farmers. The farmers work the soil, plant seasonal crops, harvest and share with members. Memberships could be a monetary contribution and/or time volunteered at a local farm or farmers market. Soil health is so important because with nutrient and microbe rich, healthy soil, you produce nutrient dense food. If done correctly, these farmers are providing the highest quality, most nutrient dense vegetables and fruits available to us. I have never tasted vegetables as fresh and nutrient dense and coming right from the farm.

Source local meats too! Find local animal farms, a neighbor that has the most beautiful chicken eggs, or local meat delivery.

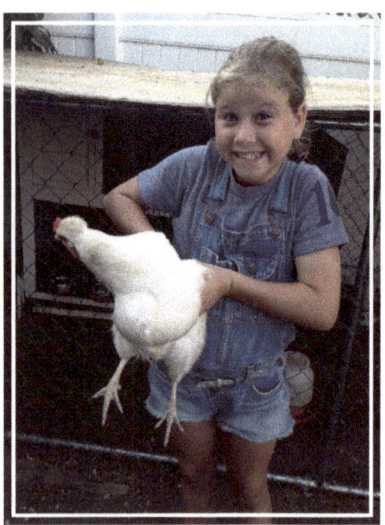 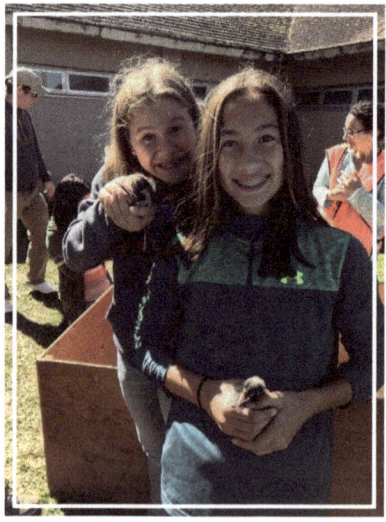 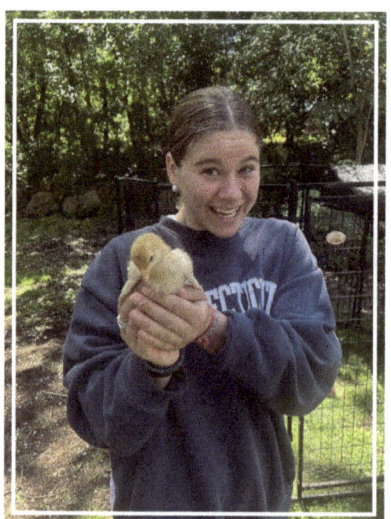

Some things don't change

We also love local fish and oysters, loaded with Zinc and Vitamin B12, is one of the most nutrient dense foods there is! Fresh Striped Bass that my husband, Bill, catches is one of life's greatest pleasures.

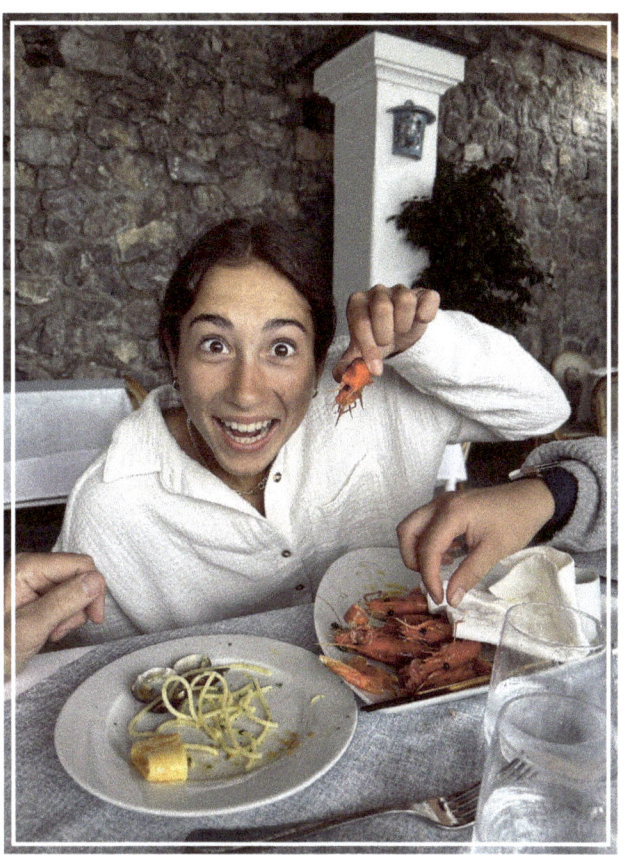

For seafood check out this link to see what and where to source your fish-
https://www.seafoodwatch.org/
There are several meat delivery services that may not be as local, but way better for your health than what you can find in your grocery store.

- Look up CSA in your area, It's worth the investment.
- Search for local farmers markets with your zip code.
- Check out: LocalHarvest.com and Eatwild.com

Some great documentaries on this topic:

"The Biggest Little Farm," directed by John Chester, Neon Films, 2019
Rotten. Directed by [Director's Name], Netflix, 2018.
"The Game Changers," directed by Louie Psihoyos, Production Company, 2018, Netflix
"The Magic Pill" 2017.
"Down to Earth with Zac Efron" (2020), directed by [Director's name], Netflix.
"The Sacred Cow". Directed by Diana Rodgers, and produced by Robb Wolf, Sacred Cow, LLC, 2020.

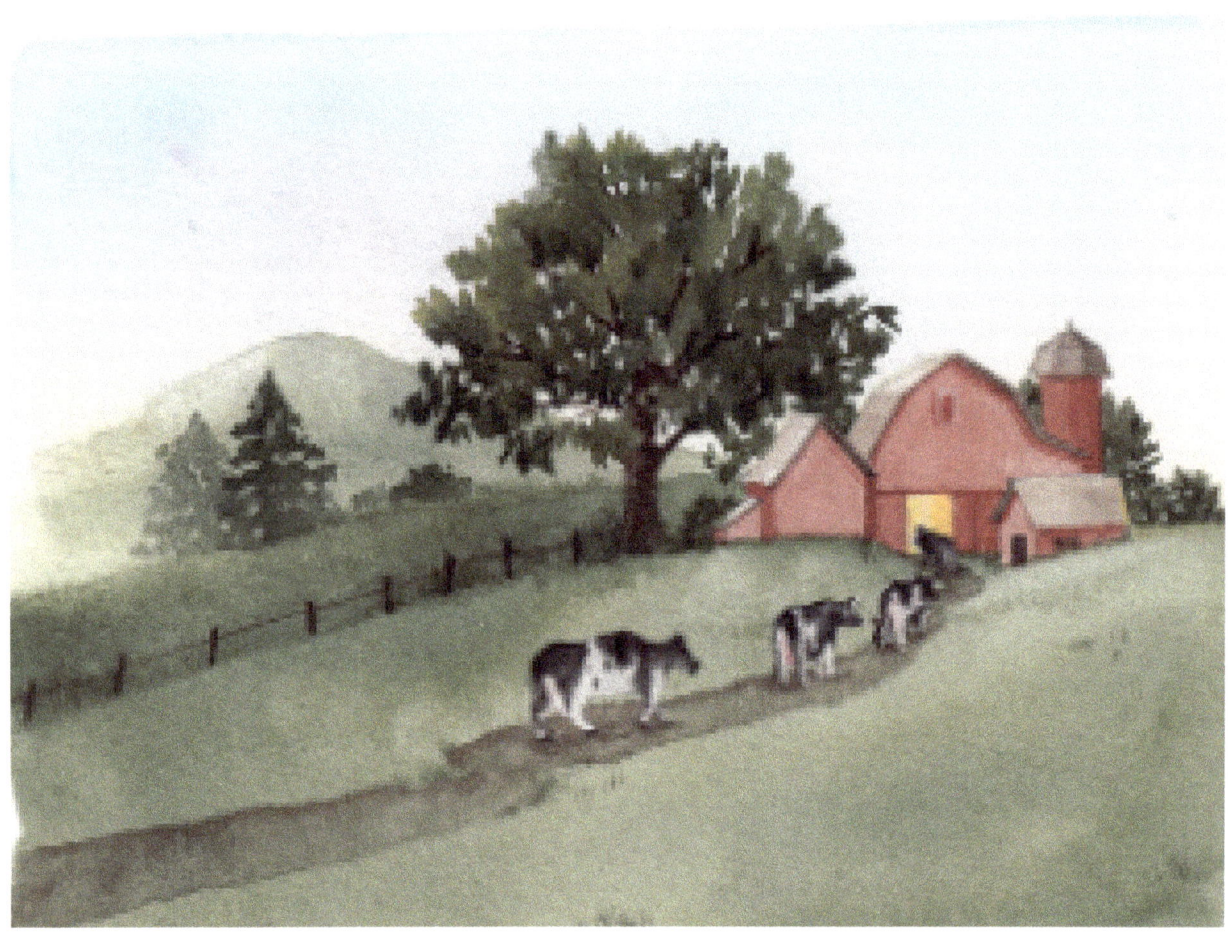

KEEP YOUR FOOD STANDARDS HIGH

HOW TO BUILD A HEALTHY PLATE FOR EACH MEAL

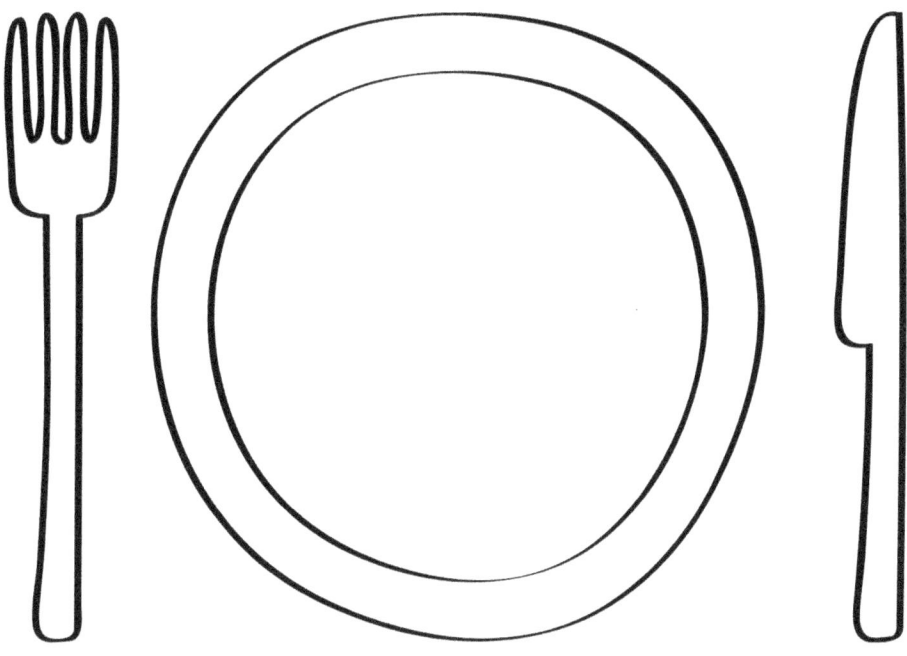

Let's get to it: Here's the *Food is My Religion* recipe for success for most meals, I do not believe there is a ONE SIZE FITS ALL model, but here's a great plan to prioritize great health, there's some flexibility here depending on where you are on your own health scale. It's important to remember that everyone is different, what works for someone else may not work for you and what works for you, may not work for someone else. Consider this an overall great guide:

Fill half of your plate with vegetables, aim to eat the rainbow, include fruit and have fun experimenting with as many colors as you can.

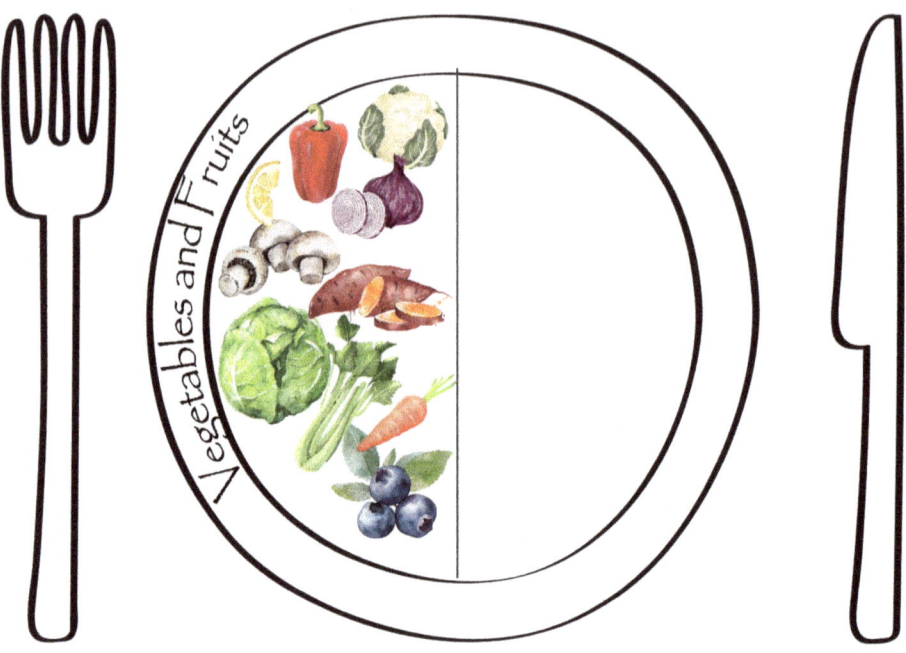

Add a palm size of protein, aim for 30 grams

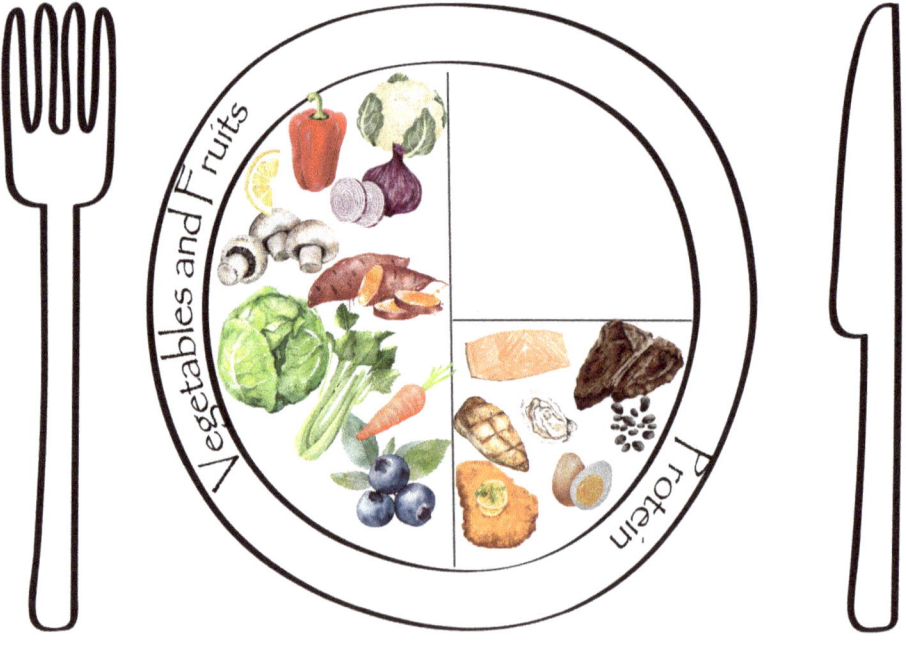

A serving of healthy fat. Remember the thumb rule.

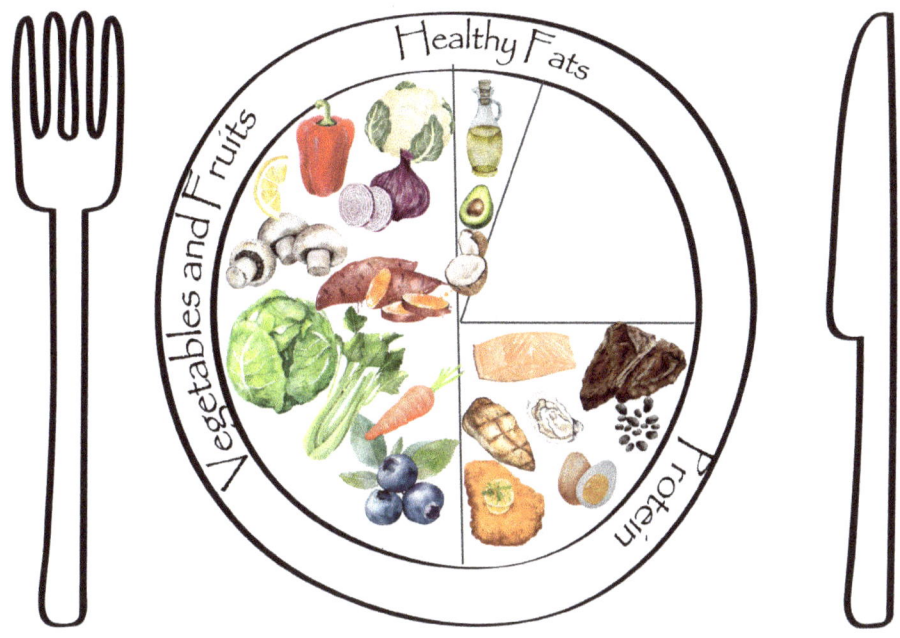

A serving of great grains

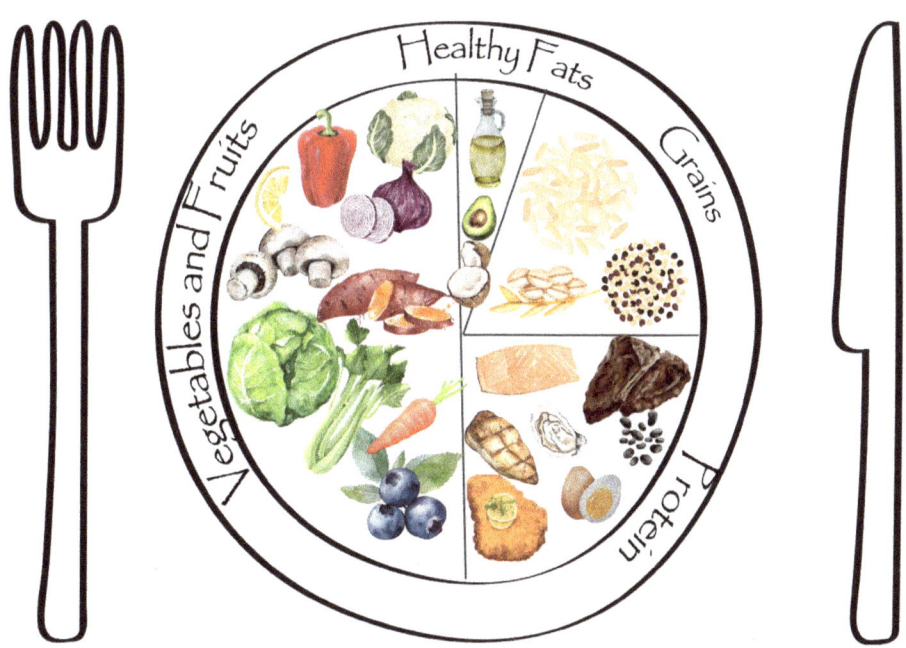

THE YES LIST

That's a great meal. And the plan I personally use 90% of the time.

If you are not lactose intolerant, try Organic Greek Yogurt and Cheeses…enjoy it in moderation. Studies also show dairy can be inflammatory, in my opinion, a good chunk of parmesan cheese or an organic goat cheese can be much healthier than the "fake cheese" labeled vegan.

Three meals of real food is a love letter to yourself.

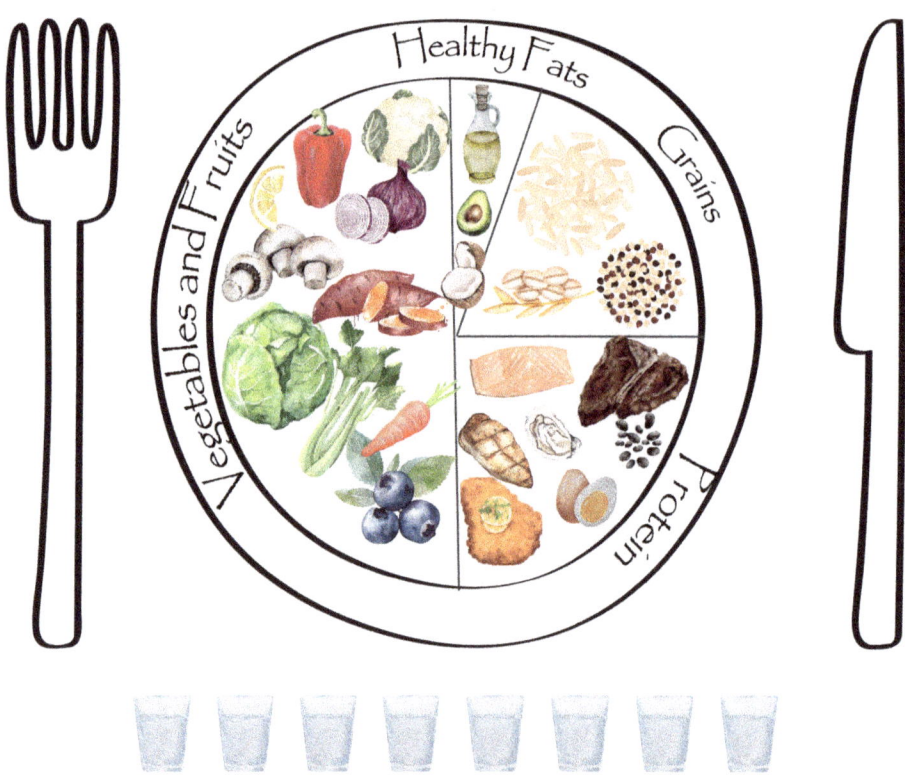

I believe food is holy—what we eat shapes every cell, every thought, every breath.

333

In my experience, it only takes 3 days to begin retraining your taste buds. Just three days! If you've been stuck in the pattern of the SAD (Standard American Diet)—heavy on processed foods, sugar, and salt—your palate has likely been overstimulated and desensitized to the natural flavors of real, whole foods. But the good news? Your taste buds can adapt faster than you think.

- In just 3 days, you can start to notice and enjoy the natural sweetness of fruits, the richness of fresh vegetables, and the satisfying flavors of whole, unprocessed foods.

- After 3 weeks, your body will begin to respond—you'll likely feel lighter, have more energy, improved digestion, and even fewer cravings for junk foods.

- By 3 months, the changes will become undeniable. Not only will you feel transformed, but the people around you will start to notice differences in your energy, skin, and overall health. Your glow will speak for itself,

This simple 3-day, 3-week, 3-month progression shows how quickly your body and mind can shift when you fuel them with what they truly need. Treat food as sacred, and it will return the favor.

Three whole days! What if you start now?

Can you commit to that and stick to it?

I believe in you.

THE NAUGHTY LIST - INGREDIENTS TO AVOID

While we focus on eating the most unprocessed foods we can, there is a time when we turn to the grocery store to buy a can of beans, loaf of bread, or a bottle of ketchup.

This generation is the first time in history that is projected to have a shorter lifespan than their parents, and this is mostly attributed to nutrition. Processed foods are killing us at alarming rates. Limiting consumption of each of these ingredients will contribute to a healthier lifestyle. Use this list to determine what products are minimally processed, and what ingredients to avoid.

The results, a deep dive into the many healthier substitutions. *As with any food ingredient, it is recommended to consult with a healthcare professional or registered dietitian if you have concerns about its consumption and its potential impact on your health.*

In efforts to keep this lighthearted, I am keeping it simple here, so use my references in the back of the book if you want more detailed information.

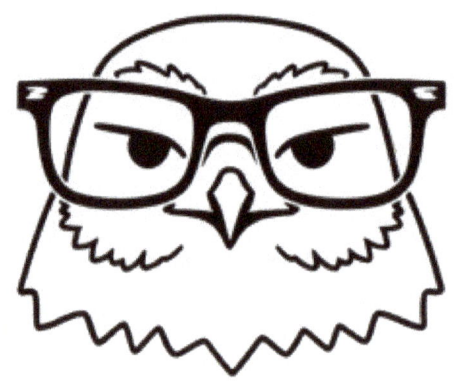

Read your labels like a hawk.

Bring this list to the grocery store when selecting your precious items. I have created a downloadable sheet for you:
https://landofnutrition.com/FIMR

Sweeteners

- REFINED SUGAR (Brown Sugar, Confectioner's Sugar, Corn Syrup, Dextrose, Fructose, Glucose, Invert Sugar, Lactose, or Milk Sugar, Levulose, Malitol, Mannitol, Raw Sugar, Sorbitol, Sucrose (table Sugar), Turbinado Sugar, Xylitol (a naturally occurring sugar in fruits but sometimes created in a lab))
- ARTIFICIAL SWEETENERS (Acesulfame potassium (Ace-K), Advantame, Alitame, Aspartame, Cyclamate, Erythritol, Hydrogenated starch hydrolysates (HSH), Isomalt, Isomaltulose, Lactitol, Maltitol, Mannitol, Neotame, Saccharin, Sorbitol, Sucralose, Xylitol)
- HIGH FRUCTOSE CORN SYRUP (HFCS)

Preservatives

- BUTYLATED HYDROXYANISOLE (BHA) & BUTYLATED HYDROXYTOLUENE (BHT)
- SODIUM NITRATE AND NITRITE
- SULFITES (Sulfur Dioxide, Sodium Sulfite, Sodium Bisulfite, Sodium Metabisulfite, Potassium Bisulfite, Potassium Metabisulfite)

Emulsifiers

- CARRAGEENAN
- CORNSTARCH
- SOY LECITHIN

Unhealthy Fats and Oils

Trans Fats (Anything Partially Hydrogenated)
- Industrial seed and vegetable oils like soybean, corn, cottonseed, safflower, sunflower, and refined canola, as well as partially hydrogenated oils (trans fats), margarine, shortening, and generic "vegetable oil" blends

Other

- ARTIFICIAL COLORS and FLAVORS
- MALTODEXTRIN
- MONOSODIUM GLUTAMATE (MSG)
- Honorable Mention -GENETICALLY MODIFIED ORGANISMS (GMOS)

SWEETENERS

REFINED SUGAR (Brown Sugar, Confectioner's Sugar, Corn Syrup, Dextrose, Fructose, Glucose, Invert Sugar, Lactose, or Milk Sugar, Levulose, Malitol, Mannitol, Raw Sugar, Sorbitol, Sucrose (table Sugar), Turbinado Sugar, Xylitol (a naturally occurring sugar in fruits but some-times created in a lab))

This is a big one, as sugar addiction is nothing to joke about - awareness is key, remember small steps result in lasting change. Trying to eliminate sugar all at once is unrealistic. If you find yourself in a sugar spiral, remember to start out slowly.

Set small goals for yourself and know that avoiding these ingredients is worth it for your health. Being mindful of your overall sugar intake (even the healthy substitutes) can help reduce the consumption of refined sugars to promote better overall health and well-being.

Why it's on the Naughty List:

- Increased Risk of Obesity
- Blood Sugar Imbalances
- Dental Health Concerns
- Inflammation and Chronic Diseases
- Nutritional Deficiencies
- Addictive Properties

Found in:

- Baked Goods
- Sodas and Sweetened Beverages
- Candies and Sweets
- Desserts
- Packaged Snacks
- Sauces and Condiments
- Processed Foods
- Medications
- Flavored Yogurts
- Bread and Baked Goods
- Canned and Packaged Foods
- Breakfast Cereals
- Flavored Coffee Drinks

ARTIFICIAL SWEETENERS (Acesulfame potassium (Ace-K), Advantame, Alitame, Aspartame, Cyclamate, Erythritol, Hydrogenated starch hydrolysates (HSH), Isomalt, Isomaltulose, Lactitol, Maltitol, Mannitol, Neotame, Saccharin, Sorbitol, Sucralose, Xylitol)

Artificial sweeteners are synthetic sugar substitutes that are designed to provide a sweet taste without the added calories of regular sugar. While they can be beneficial for individuals looking to reduce their calorie intake or manage diabetes, there are several concerns associated with their use that have led to questions about their overall safety.

Why it's on the Naughty List

- Impact on Metabolic Health: Your body's ability to efficiently use the foods you eat for energy and dispose of what is not needed. Risks of Insulin Resistance and Type 2 Diabetes, High blood pressure, high cholesterol, weight gain.
- Potential for Increased Sweet Cravings and Negative Impact on Taste Perception: Leading to a higher overall calorie intake and a greater likelihood of developing a preference for highly processed, sugary foods.
- Association with Health Risks, Neurological effects and an increased risk of certain cancers.
- Impact on Gut Health

Found In:

- Diet Sodas and carbonated beverages
- Low-Calorie or Sugar-Free Snacks-Sugar-Free Condiments and Sauces
- Baked Goods and Desserts
- Packaged Foods and Snack Bars
- Medications and Supplements

HIGH FRUCTOSE CORN SYRUP (HFCS)

High fructose corn syrup (HFCS) is a sweetener derived from cornstarch, which is also an emulsifier, and is commonly used in a wide range of processed foods and beverages. The consumption of HFCS has increased significantly over the past few decades (as has heart disease), there are concerns about its potential health effects, which have led to questions about its overall safety.

Why it's on the Naughty List:

- Increased Risk of Obesity
- Impact on Metabolic Health: -Risks of Insulin Resistance and Type 2 Diabetes, High blood pressure, high cholesterol, and insulin resistance: Your body's ability to efficiently use the foods you eat for energy and dispose of what is not needed.

- ✕ Liver Health
- ✕ Appetite Regulation

Found in:

- ✕ Soft Drinks and Sodas
- ✕ Packaged Foods
- ✕ Baked Goods
- ✕ Condiments and Sauces
- ✕ Breakfast Cereals and Cereal Bars
- ✕ Desserts and Snack Foods

Healthier Options SWEETENERS

Good News: There are several natural sweeteners available that can be used in place of refined and artificial sugars to add sweetness to your dishes and beverages. When choosing natural sweeteners, it is essential to be mindful of portion sizes and overall sugar intake, as excessive consumption of any sweetener, natural or artificial, can still have negative health effects. Incorporating these natural alternatives in moderation can help reduce your overall sugar intake while still satisfying your sweet tooth, all in moderation. Nonetheless, it is crucial to consult with a healthcare professional before making any significant dietary changes or using artificial sweeteners regularly, especially for individuals with pre-existing health conditions.

Some healthy alternatives to refined sugar include:

- ✓ Stevia: Derived from the leaves of the Stevia rebaudiana plant. It is much sweeter than sugar, has no calories making it a popular alternative for those looking to reduce calorie intake.
- ✓ Raw Honey: High in antioxidant, antibacterial and antifungal properties. Not to be given to children under 1 year old.
- ✓ 100% Pure Maple Syrup: From the sap of maple trees. It contains various antioxidants and minerals. Great as a healthier alternative in pancakes, waffles, and desserts.
- ✓ Coconut Sugar: (Not coconut palm sugar) Derived from the sap of the coconut palm tree, contains some nutrients such as iron, zinc, and antioxidants. Substitute 1:1 in baking and cooking.
- ✓ Molasses: A byproduct of the sugar refining process and contains various vitamins and minerals, including iron, calcium, and potassium, providing a rich, caramel-like flavor.
- ✓ Dates and Date Paste: Provides natural sweetness and a rich, caramel-like flavor. Eat whole Dates for a sweet natural snack or blend to make a paste to sweeten baked goods.

- ✓ Agave Nectar: Has a lower glycemic index than sugar alone. Use in moderation.
- ✓ Fruit Purees: Applesauce, banana puree, and other fruit purees can be used as natural sweeteners and substitutes in various recipes, including baked goods and desserts.
- ✓ Monk Fruit Extract: Also known as Luo Han Guo. It is a zero-calorie sweetener that can be used as a sugar substitute in various food and beverage products.

PRESERVATIVES

BUTYLATED HYDROXYANISOLE (BHA) & BUTYLATED HYDROXYTOLUENE (BHT)

Butylated hydroxyanisole (BHA) and butylated hydroxytoluene (BHT) are synthetic antioxidants that are commonly used as preservatives to prolong shelf life in a wide range of food and personal care products. While they have been approved for use by regulatory authorities, including the U.S. Food and Drug Administration (FDA), concerns have been raised about their potential health risks.

Why it's on the Naughty List:

- ✗ Carcinogenic Potential
- ✗ Endocrine Disruption
- ✗ Allergic Reactions
- ✗ Potential Toxicity
- ✗ Environmental Concerns

Found In:

- ✗ Packaged Foods
- ✗ Cosmetics and Personal Care Products
- ✗ Medications and Supplements
- ✗ Pet Food
- ✗ Packaging Materials

SODIUM NITRATE AND NITRITE

Sodium nitrate and sodium nitrite are preservatives used in processed meats such as bacon, ham, hot dogs, and deli meats to prevent the growth of harmful bacteria and improve shelf life.. While their use has been approved by regulatory agencies, concerns have been raised about their potential health effects.

It's best to choose fresh unprocessed meats, those without sodium nitrate and sodium nitrite, incorporating a variety of whole foods into your diet lowers potential health risks associated with their consumption.

Why it's on the Naughty List:

- Formation of Nitrosamines, potential carcinogenic compounds
- Impact on Cardiovascular Health
- Potential for Allergic Reactions
- Infant Health Concerns

Found in:

- Processed Meats
- Canned Meats
- Smoked and Fermented Meats
- Jerky and Dried Meat Snacks
- Cured Fish Products

SULFITES (Sulfur Dioxide, Sodium Sulfite, Sodium Bisulfite, Sodium Metabisulfite, Potassium Bisulfite, Potassium Metabisulfite)

Sulfites are sulfur-based compounds that occur naturally in some foods and are also used as additives in various processed foods and beverages to prevent discoloration, inhibit microbial growth, and extend shelf life. Some individuals may be sensitive to sulfites and experience adverse allergenic or gastrointestinal reactions after consuming foods or beverages containing these additives.

Why it's on the Naughty List:

- Allergic Reactions
- Asthma Exacerbation
- Gastrointestinal Distress
- Potential for Toxicity

Found In:

- Processed Foods, especially Meats
- Condiments and Pickled Foods and relishes
- Dried Fruits and Vegetables
- Wine and Beer
- Baked Goods
- Canned and Frozen Seafood
- Prepared Soups and Broths

Healthier Options PRESERVATIVES

There are several natural and safer options available which can help extend the shelf life of products without the potential health risks associated with synthetic preservatives. By using these natural alternatives and methods, you can reduce your reliance on synthetic preservatives. It's important to understand the specific properties and uses of each alternative to ensure successful substitution and to maintain food safety and quality. By using these natural alternatives and methods, manufacturers can create products that are safer and healthier for consumers, while still maintaining product quality and extending shelf life.

- ✓ Natural Curing Alternatives: Celery juice, which naturally contains nitrates, or sea salt to preserve and flavor meats.

- ✓ Herbs and Spices: Garlic, ginger, and cloves contain natural antimicrobial properties, prevent food spoilage and enhance the flavor of your dishes. Rosemary extract is a natural antioxidant that can be used as a preservative in food products, cosmetics, and personal care items. It has antimicrobial properties and can help prevent the growth of microorganisms..

- ✓ Salt: A natural preservative in curing and pickling processes to inhibit the growth of bacteria and extend the shelf life of foods, especially in meat, fish, and vegetable preservation.

- ✓ Vinegar and Citrus Juices: Flavor enhancers great for marinades and dressings to prolong the shelf life of foods and add a tangy taste.

- ✓ Natural Fermentation: Utilize natural fermentation processes (see Sauerkraut recipe in Part 2) to preserve and flavor foods, such as fermented vegetables and cultured dairy products, which can provide beneficial probiotics and natural preservation without the need for synthetic preservatives.

- ✓ Ascorbic Acid (Vitamin C): Ascorbic acid, or vitamin C, is a natural antioxidant that can be used, it helps prevent the oxidation of foods and can also be used to maintain the color and freshness of certain products.

- ✓ Vitamin E (Tocopherol): Natural antioxidant that can be used helps prevent the oxidation of fats and oils, thereby extending the shelf life of these products.

- ✓ Green Tea Extract: Natural antioxidants have antimicrobial properties and can help prevent the growth of bacteria and fungi, extending the shelf life of these products. Look for Camellia sinensis, GTE, Epigallocatechin gallate (EGCG), also known as epigallocatechin-3-gallate or Green Tea Catechins.

- ✓ Citric Acid: Commonly found in citrus fruits and can help enhance the flavor and stability of foods.

- ✓ Grapeseed Extract: Antimicrobial properties and can help prevent the growth of microorganisms, thereby extending the shelf life of these products.
- ✓ Proper Storage Techniques: Store foods properly by refrigerating or freezing them at appropriate temperatures to slow down the growth of bacteria and maintain their freshness and quality without the need for chemical preservatives.

EMULSIFIERS
CARRAGEENAN

Carrageenan is a very common food additive derived from red seaweed and is often used as a thickening or stabilizing agent to improve texture, consistency, and shelf life in a variety of processed foods and dairy products. While it has been deemed safe for consumption by regulatory agencies such as the U.S. Food and Drug Administration (FDA) and the European Food Safety Authority (EFSA), concerns have been raised about its potential health effects, including a higher risk of cancer. A NEW STUDY IN FRANCE, found that certain emulsifiers (thickening and preserving ingredients) can increase the risk of cancer up to 46% and 32% higher risk of breast cancer in women who often eat products with Carrageenan.

Why risk it?

Despite these concerns, carrageenan is still commonly used in the food industry (and can easily be found at Health Food Stores). Some food manufacturers have started to replace carrageenan with other stabilizers and thickeners, such as guar gum, locust bean gum, and xanthan gum, to address these potential health risks. As with any food additive, it is important for consumers to be aware of potential sensitivities or adverse reactions and to consume carrageenan-containing products in moderation.

Why it's on the Naughty List:

- ✗ Potential Cancer Risk*
- ✗ Gastrointestinal Issues
- ✗ Allergic Reactions
- ✗ Inflammatory Response
- ✗ Disruption of Gut Microbiota: by now, you should know how important your microbiome and healthy gut flora is.

Found In:

- Dairy Products
- Processed Meats
- Plant-Based Milk Alternatives
- Desserts and Puddings
- Confectionery
- Pet Food, particularly in wet pet food formulations.

CORNSTARCH

Cornstarch, a common thickening agent derived from corn, is generally considered safe for consumption and is widely used in various culinary applications. However, there are some potential concerns associated with its use, especially when consumed in large quantities or by individuals with specific dietary considerations.

Why it's on the Naughty List:

- High Glycemic Index
- Caloric Content
- Potential Allergens
- Processing Concerns
- Digestive Issues

Found in:

- Baked Goods
- Sauces, Gravies and Soups
- Desserts
- Fried Foods
- Dairy Products
- Processed Foods

SOY LECITHIN

Soy lecithin, another unfortunate common additive, is a byproduct of the soybean oil production process and is commonly used as an emulsifier in various food products and as an ingredient in supplements and medications. Individuals with soy allergies or sensitivities should be cautious when consuming products containing soy lecithin and may need to avoid them to prevent allergic reactions.

Why it's on the Naughty List:

- ✗ Allergies and Sensitivities
- ✗ Genetically Modified Source
- ✗ Phytoestrogens
- ✗ Processing Concerns

Found In:

- ✗ Chocolates and Confectionery
- ✗ Baked Goods
- ✗ Dairy Products
- ✗ Processed Foods
- ✗ Nutritional Supplements & Vitamins
- ✗ Pharmaceuticals
- ✗ Cosmetics and Personal Care Products

Healthier Options EMULSIFIERS:

There are several natural options that can be used as thickeners and stabilizers that can help maintain the texture and stability of foods without the potential health risks. Food manufacturers can create products that are safer and healthier for consumers, while still maintaining the desired texture and stability. Additionally, consumers can make more informed choices by selecting products that contain natural thickeners and stabilizers, thereby reducing their exposure to potentially harmful additives.

Some of these alternatives include:

- ✓ **Guar Gum:** A natural fiber derived from guar beans commonly used in various food products, including baked goods, dairy products, and sauces, to improve texture and stability, particularly in gluten-free and vegan baking.
- ✓ **Locust Bean Gum:** Also known as carob gum, is a natural thickening and stabilizing agent derived from the seeds of the carob tree. It is often used as a carrageenan alternative in dairy products, ice creams, and other food products.
- ✓ **Sunflower Lecithin:** Derived from sunflower seeds, can be used as an alternative to soy lecithin in baked goods, chocolates, and dressings.
- ✓ **Egg Yolks:** Commonly used in cooking and baking to create smooth and creamy textures in sauces, dressings, and desserts.
- ✓ **Xanthan Gum:** Can help improve the texture and shelf life of foods without the potential health risks, particularly in gluten free baking.

- ✓ Agar-Agar: A safer natural gelling agent derived from seaweed. It is often used as a vegetarian alternative to gelatin.
- ✓ Arrowroot: A gluten free starchy substance derived from the roots of several tropical plants. It works as an excellent thickening agent and can be used as a one-to-one replacement for cornstarch in most recipes. I love baking with this easily accessible powder.
- ✓ Tapioca Starch: Tapioca starch is derived from the cassava root. It has a similar texture to cornstarch, without the negative effects.
- ✓ Potato Starch: Derived from potatoes, a versatile thickening agent that can be used in both sweet and savory dishes.
- ✓ Rice Flour: Made from finely milled rice.
- ✓ Chia Seeds or Flaxseeds: Chia seeds and flaxseeds can be used as natural thickeners in some recipes, especially in puddings, jams, and sauces (see recipe for Chia Jam in Part 2). They provide additional nutritional benefits, including fiber and essential fatty acids. Powerhouse ingredients with multiple nutrition benefits.

UNHEALTHY FATS AND OILS

TRANS FATS (ANYTHING PARTIALLY HYDROGENATED)

Industrial Seed and Vegetable Oils (Corn, Cottonseed, Generic "Vegetable Oil" Blends, Margarine, Partially Hydrogenated Oils (Trans Fats), Refined Canola, Safflower, Shortening, Soybean, Sunflower)

These oils are heavily processed, often with chemical solvents and high heat, making them prone to oxidation and harmful compounds that fuel inflammation, heart disease, and other chronic illnesses. Instead, choose healthier, stable fats like extra virgin olive oil, avocado oil, coconut oil, or ghee.

Trans fats are a type of unsaturated fatty acid that have been partially hydrogenated to improve the shelf life and stability of processed foods. While naturally occurring trans fats can be found in small amounts in some animal products, partially hydrogenated trans fats, commonly found in processed foods, have been linked to various health concerns.

Due to the detrimental health effects associated with the consumption of trans fats, many countries have implemented regulations to reduce or eliminate the use of partially hydrogenated oils in food production, and the United States is catching on. Due to the health risks associated with the consumption of trans fats, many health organizations and regulatory bodies have implemented measures to reduce their presence in the food supply. Checking food labels and avoiding products containing partially hydrogenated oils can help minimize the intake of trans fats and promote better overall health and well-being. Packaged Food Labels in the USA are required to list Trans Fat.

Why it's on the Naughty List:

- Increased Risk of Heart Disease: Shown to increase levels of LDL (bad) cholesterol and decrease levels of HDL (good) cholesterol, leading to an increased risk of heart disease, stroke, and other cardiovascular problems.
- Inflammation and Chronic Diseases: Associated with the development of chronic diseases such as diabetes, obesity, and certain types of cancer.
- Adverse Effects on Blood Vessels: Can have detrimental effects on blood vessels, leading to reduced flexibility and impaired function, which can contribute to an increased risk of heart disease and other cardiovascular complications.
- Negative Impact on Metabolic Health: Linked to insulin resistance, metabolic syndrome, and an increased risk of developing type 2 diabetes, which can have far-reaching implications for overall health and well-being.
- Brain Health Concerns: Associated with an increased risk of neurodegenerative diseases and cognitive decline, highlighting potential concerns regarding brain health and function.

Found In:

- Packaged Snacks
- Fried Foods
- Baked Goods
- Margarine and Shortening
- Fast Food
- Packaged Ready-to-Eat Meals: Microwave Popcorn, non-dairy creamers, frozen pizza for example.
- Amusement Parks and some school lunches

Healthier Options FATS AND OILS

Consume in moderation, remember serving sizes and rule of thumb (use your thumb as a serving size of healthy fats).

- ✓ Extra virgin olive oil: A healthy source of monounsaturated fats and can be used for cooking, sautéing, and salad dressings as a substitute for trans fats. (Best raw or for cooking at low temperatures.)
- ✓ Avocado Oil: Rich in monounsaturated fats and has a high smoke point, making it suitable for high-heat cooking methods such as frying and grilling.
- ✓ Nuts and Seeds: Incorporating natural sources of fats from nuts and seeds, such as almonds, walnuts, and flaxseeds, into your diet can provide healthy fats and essential nutrients without the harmful effects of trans fats.
- ✓ Fatty Fish: Consuming fatty fish such as salmon, mackerel, and trout provides omega-3 fatty acids, which are beneficial for heart health and can serve as a healthier alternative to trans fats.
- ✓ Nut Butters: Natural nut butters, such as almond butter and peanut butter, can be used as spreads and ingredients in recipes to add healthy fats and protein without the negative effects of trans fats and industrial oils.

OTHER

ARTIFICIAL COLORS AND FLAVORS

Food manufacturers add artificial flavors and colors to "enhance" taste and appearance and to make them more visually appealing and flavorful. Unprocessed and whole ingredients can help in avoiding artificial flavors and colors. Fresh fruits, vegetables, whole grains, and natural sweeteners can provide natural flavors and colors to foods and beverages.

Don't get fooled.

Why it's on the Naughty List

- ✗ Multiple Health Risks: Hyperactivity, Allergic reactions. Studies show Red 3 causes cancer in Lab Animals, and others are also carcinogenic
- ✗ Allergic Reactions: Leading to symptoms such as hives, itching, or respiratory problems.

- ✗ No Nutritional Value: May mean that you're consuming more empty calories without any beneficial nutrients.
- ✗ Misleading Perception: Masking the natural qualities of food, leading consumers to perceive products as more nutritious or flavorful than they actually are. This can result in poor dietary choices and an over reliance on processed foods.
- ✗ Environmental Impact: The production of artificial colors and flavors often involves the use of synthetic chemicals and can contribute to environmental pollution if not managed properly.

Found in:

- ✗ Processed food: Snacks, candies, baked goods, cereals, chips, sauces, condiments
- ✗ Beverages: Sodas, fruit drinks, energy drinks, flavored beverages
- ✗ Convenience Foods: Ready-to-eat meals, instant noodles, frozen dinners, and other convenience foods
- ✗ Medications and Supplements: Can be added to make them more palatable or visually appealing.
- ✗ Cosmetics and Personal Care Products: Cosmetics, skincare products, toothpaste, and other personal care

Healthier Options ARTIFICIAL COLORS AND FLAVORS

- ✓ Natural Food Coloring derived from various plant sources such as fruits, vegetables, and spices. Beets can be used to create a red or pink color, turmeric can produce yellow, and spirulina, a type of algae with significant health benefits, can create blue and green hues. Have fun!
- ✓ Herbs and spices can be used to add natural flavors to foods and beverages. Cinnamon, vanilla, ginger, and mint can add a rich flavor without the need for artificial additives. Saffron, annatto, and paprika can be used as natural colorants that can provide vibrant colors and flavors to a wide range of food products.
- ✓ Fruit and vegetable juices can be used to provide both color and flavor
- ✓ Natural Flavor Extracts such as those derived from fruits, nuts, and seeds, can be used to enhance the taste of food and beverages.

MONOSODIUM GLUTAMATE (MSG)

Monosodium glutamate (MSG) is a flavor enhancer commonly used in various processed and restaurant (note Chinese food and soup stands) foods to improve the overall taste and flavor profile of dishes. Some individuals may experience adverse reactions after consuming foods containing MSG. There was a certain soup chain restaurant that we would often go to, it took a while to make the association that I would get a headache after this meal, but I realized it was the MSG that was causing it! A reminder to pay attention to the signals from your body.

While the FDA considers MSG to be generally recognized as safe (GRAS) for consumption, some individuals experience a response known as "Chinese restaurant syndrome" or MSG symptom complex.

To minimize potential risks, look for foods labeled as "MSG-free," call ahead or choose whole, unprocessed foods that do not contain added MSG. It is important to consult a healthcare professional if you experience severe or persistent symptoms after consuming foods containing MSG.

Why it's on the Naughty List:

- Adverse Reactions: Headaches, sweating, flushing
- Sensitivity and Allergies: Skin rashes, itching, or respiratory problems
- Potential Health Effects: Such as metabolic disorders, neurological effects, and weight gain.

Found in:

- Packaged Foods
- Soups and Broths
- Fast Food and Restaurant Dishes: Best practice is to call ahead or check menus online.
- Sauces and Seasonings: Soy sauce, teriyaki sauce, and certain seasoning blends.
- Processed Meats and Snack Foods
- Flavor Enhancers and Condiments

Healthier Options MSG

- ✓ Herbs and Spices: Basil, cilantro, oregano, thyme, and rosemary, to add natural flavors and aromas to your dishes.
- ✓ Citrus Juices and Zests: Use freshly squeezed citrus juices and zests, such as lemon, lime, and orange to add brightness and tanginess to your dishes without the need for artificial flavor enhancers.
- ✓ Aromatics: Utilize aromatics like garlic, ginger, and onions to add depth and savory notes to your dishes, creating a rich and flavorful base for your cooking.
- ✓ Natural Umami (fancy word for savory) Tomatoes, mushrooms, and seaweed (look for nori and furikake to sprinkle) to enhance the savory taste of your soups and dishes and provide a natural alternative to MSG.
- ✓ Homemade Broths and Stocks: Prepare homemade broths and stocks using fresh vegetables, herbs, and quality meat or bones to create a flavorful base for soups, stews, and sauces, without the need for added flavor enhancers.
- ✓ Fermented Products: Incorporate fermented products such as miso, organic low sodium soy sauce, tamari, coconut aminos (my favorite) and fermented bean pastes to add complex and savory flavors to your dishes, providing a natural umami taste without the use of artificial additives.

MALTODEXTRIN

When reading ingredient labels, maltodextrin may appear under its own name or as part of a compound ingredient. A highly processed ingredient derived from starch, typically corn, rice, or potato. We are trying to avoid heavily processed foods and ingredients in favor of whole, natural alternatives.

This malicious ingredient can be found also as an emulsifier, but also as a sweetening agent.

Why it's on the Naughty List:

- ✗ High Glycemic Index: Can cause a rapid spike in blood sugar levels when consumed. For people with diabetes or those trying to manage their blood sugar levels, this rapid increase can be problematic.
- ✗ Empty Calories: It provides energy but lacks significant nutritional value.
- ✗ Potential for Digestive Issues

- × Processed Nature:
- × Not Suitable for Some Dietary Restrictions for it's high carbohydrate content.

Found in:

- × Processed Foods:
- × Snack foods: Baked goods (cookies, cakes, pastries), breakfast cereals, instant pudding mixes, salad dressings, instant soups and sauces.
- × Beverages: Powdered drink mixes, sports drinks
- × Convenience Foods: Ready-to-eat meals, frozen dinners, and canned goods
- × Dietary Supplements: Vitamins, minerals, and protein powders
- × Medications: Pharmaceutical formulations
- × Baby Formulas

Healthier Options MALTODEXTRIN

- ✓ Whole Food Thickeners: Mashed fruits (like bananas or applesauce), pureed vegetables (such as sweet potatoes or cauliflower), or chia seeds, white beans are great for soups and stews.
- ✓ Whole Grains: Whole grains like quinoa, brown rice, oats, and barley provide fiber, vitamins, and minerals in addition to carbohydrates.
- ✓ Natural Starches: Arrowroot powder and tapioca flour,
- ✓ Fruit Powders: Fruit powders made from dried fruits like berries, mangoes, or apples can add flavor and natural sweetness.
- ✓ Low Glycemic Index Sweeteners: Coconut sugar, monk fruit sweetener, or stevia.
- ✓ Nutritional Yeast: A great savory flavor enhancer and thickener in recipes, providing a cheesy or nutty taste along with a range of nutrients like B vitamins and protein.
- ✓ Inulin: A prebiotic fiber found naturally in some foods like chicory root. It can be used as a sweetener or thickener in certain recipes and provides additional digestive health benefits.

Honorable Mention

GENETICALLY MODIFIED ORGANISMS (GMOS)

The topic of GMOs is complex and often controversial—just ask my son, Liam, who makes some valid points. While there are concerns, it's worth weighing the scientific consensus and research to make your own choice.

Not all GMOs are created equal, I almost removed them from my "naughty list." For example, if rice can be modified to resist drought, it could fight food scarcity, that is a positive. But when crops are engineered to survive via toxic pesticides, glyphosate particularly, it means those chemicals end up in our soil, on our food, and eventually in our bodies. The effects of inviting more poison into our food and environment are detrimental and several studies show evidence enough to avoid.

Why it's on the List:

- Potential Allergies & Toxicity: Liver and kidney damage, inflammation, and reproductive issues
- Pesticide Residues: Crops are engineered to survive heavy pesticide spraying, leaving higher chemical residues on food, which may be harmful to human health.
- Lack of Long-Term Studies: Safety assessments are short-term and industry-funded, leaving uncertainty about chronic health effects such as cancer, endocrine disruption, and gut microbiome impacts.
- Superweeds & Superpests: Over-reliance on herbicide-tolerant GM crops has led to herbicide-resistant weeds and pesticide-resistant insects, requiring even more toxic chemicals.
- Biodiversity Loss: Monocultures reduce crop diversity, threaten pollinators and beneficial insects, potentially destabilizing ecosystems.
- Soil & Water Contamination: Increased chemical use from GMO farming contaminates soil and waterways, harming wildlife and aquatic ecosystems.
- Seed Patents: A handful of powerful biotech corporations control patented GMO seeds, forcing farmers to buy new seeds each year instead of saving them.
- Farmer Dependence: Small farmers often face legal and economic pressure if non-GMO crops are accidentally cross-pollinated by GMO varieties.
- Food Sovereignty: Critics argue GMOs erode local food systems, concentrating control of the global food supply in the hands of a few companies.

- ✗ Yields & Hunger: Studies suggest GMO crops do not consistently outperform conventional or organic methods in yield or profitability.

Found in:

- ✗ Crops and Produce: most common are corn, soybeans, cotton, canola, and some varieties of squash and papaya.
- ✗ Processed Foods: Cornstarch, corn syrup, soy lecithin, and sugar from sugar beets.
- ✗ Livestock Feed: Some animal feed contains genetically modified ingredients such as corn and soybeans
- ✗ can then be consumed by livestock, potentially resulting in animal products derived from animals raised on GMO feed. Cue "The Circle of Life"
- ✗ Medications and Supplements: Some medications and dietary supplements may contain ingredients derived from genetically modified microorganisms, such as certain enzymes and additives used in pharmaceutical and nutritional products.
- ✗ Industrial and Non-Food Products: Biofuels, fibers, and biodegradable plastics
- ✗ Agricultural Practices: GMOs are also found in various agricultural practices, including the use of genetically modified crops for research, cultivation, and experimental purposes, as well as for the production of seeds and agricultural inputs.

Healthier Options GMOS

While GMOs are present in various products and practices, it is important to note that regulations and labeling requirements for GMOs may vary by country. Consumers who wish to avoid GMOs can look for products labeled as "non-GMO" or "GMO-free" or choose organic products, which are produced without the use of genetically modified organisms. (Remember to look for the 5 digit code on produce beginning with 9 for organic).

- ✓ Organic Produce: Opt for organic fruits and vegetables that are grown without the use of genetically modified seeds or synthetic pesticides, ensuring a more natural and environmentally friendly option, see my list of where to buy organic and where you don't have to.
- ✓ Non-GMO Project Verified Products: Look for products that are Non-GMO Project Verified, indicating that they have undergone rigorous testing to ensure they are free of genetically modified ingredients.

- ✓ Certified Organic Meat and Dairy: Choose organic meat and dairy products from animals that have been raised on organic feed without the use of GMOs or synthetic hormones and antibiotics.
- ✓ Non-GMO Cooking Oils: Select cooking oils that are labeled as non-GMO, such as organic canola oil, organic sunflower oil, or organic olive oil, to avoid genetically modified ingredients.
- ✓ Whole Foods and Grains: Opt for whole foods and grains that are certified organic or labeled as non-GMO, such as organic rice, quinoa, oats, and whole wheat, to ensure you're consuming products that are free of genetically modified ingredients. You cannot go wrong here.
- ✓ Organic or Non-GMO Snacks: Choose snacks and packaged foods that are certified organic or labeled as non-GMO to avoid genetically modified ingredients and ensure you're making healthier snack choices.

"Let food be the medicine and medicine be the food"

– Hippocrates

LABEL READING IS A SPIRITUAL PRACTICE

A Few Sacred Notes on What to Eat—and What to Avoid
There's a world of difference between "processed" and the new villain in town: "ultra-processed."

Can you find healthy processed foods? Absolutely!
The magic is in knowing where to look—and reading labels like a detective on a mission.

Cracking open a can of beans is not a sin. It's a lifesaver compared to soaking and simmering for hours. For a great protein option, just look for organic beans in BPA-free cans.

The same goes for ketchup, crackers, and butter. Use the Naughty List as your sacred scroll when navigating pre-packaged foods. And let's be real—sometimes life calls for grab-and-go snacks. Nuts, seeds, and a clean beef jerky can save you from the depths of Hangry, but only if you peek at the ingredients first. (Read that label and—boom—you're a superhero.)

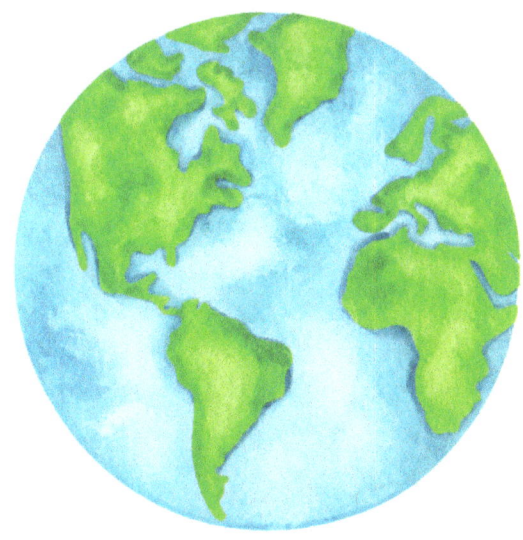

A short list of grocery brands to look for and trust:

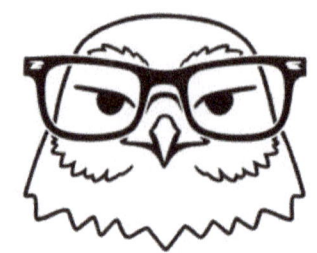

Applegate – Clean deli meats, hot dogs, and sausages

Bob's Red Mill - A variety of trustworthy baking supplies: flours, oats, cornmeal and baking soda

Chosen Foods – Avocado oils and mayo alternatives

Chomps – Grass-fed meat sticks

Epic – Meat bars and bone broth

Fourth and Heart – Grass-fed flavored ghee

Kettle and Fire – Bone broth and clean soups

Muir Glen – Organic canned tomatoes and sauces with simple ingredients

Paleo Valley - Beef sticks, bone broths, organ capsules, and bars

Primal Kitchen – Sauces, dressings, and collagen

Siete Foods – Grain-free sauces and seasonings

Vital Farms – Pasture-raised eggs and butter

RITUALS

I believe in rituals

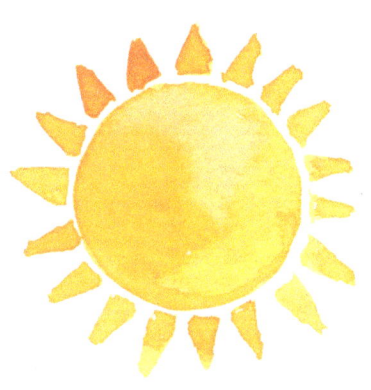

First thing in the morning, squeeze half a lemon into some warm water, step outside, or stand near a window, take all the beauty of nature in as you sip your way to a healthier you.

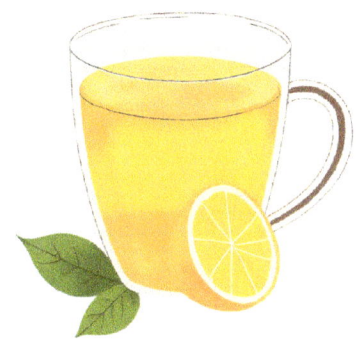

A calm mind and a nourished body are unstoppable.
This simple ritual will help you take a few moments for yourself, before you give to everyone else. Starting with water and lemon puts you in the right direction for staying hydrated for the day, helping your body to be in a good flow. Your digestive system will thank you, as this simple step will stimulate your metabolism, wake up your liver, help with bloating, prevent kidney stones and fight indigestion. Get a boost of Vitamin C, helps your body fight off infections and promotes glowing skin. Plus, the antioxidants from citrus will improve your heart health.

The sunlight on your face is another health benefit first thing in the morning, the more exposure we can get, the better your overall wellbeing can be. Regulating your body's natural circadian rhythm, the sun exposure early in the morning can boost Vitamin D, Improve your mood, stave away illnesses by boosting your immune system, improve your mental health and much more.

HERBAL TEA

This is my go-to for staving off cravings and preventing me from overeating or eating out of boredom. I have found that a "not so healthy" craving could be averted with simply brewing a cup of tea, much less calories and much more benefits of spirituality than snarfing down a bag of chips or a muffin. A daily cup of tea is like a reset button, flooding your body with plant-powered antioxidants while grounding your spirit.

There are so many herbal teas to choose from, stand in any tea section at the grocery store and just look at the variety of flavors, colors, tastes, packaging. Read your labels, choose organic, read about the source from where the tea is from and indulge in one of my favorite rituals, tea time.

Find meditation in the selection, brewing and consuming a cup of tea mid-morning and mid-afternoon. Some favorites are: Chamomile, Mint, Rooibos, Nettle leaf with 1 tsp honey (great if you are on an antibiotic). From chamomile to green tea, every leaf carries ancient medicine—anti-inflammatory, detoxifying, and deeply nourishing.

Take a deep breath, open your cabinet, select your tea with care - brew your herbal tea as directed. Use a spoon to stir, one way or another. Put intention into this moment. Give it a stir and blessing, be mindful of the act of making a cup of tea. Say a little prayer. Bonus if you use a pretty spoon to stir your intentions gently in a clockwise direction.

Herbal Tea can be so healing:

Chamomile – Promotes relaxation, improves sleep, aids digestion, reduces inflammation.

Dandelion – Supports liver health, aids digestion, natural detoxifier, rich in vitamins.

Echinacea – Boosts immune function, helps fight colds, reduces inflammation.

Ginger – Aids digestion, reduces nausea, supports immune function, and has anti-inflammatory properties.

Hibiscus – Rich in antioxidants, lowers blood pressure, supports heart health, boosts immunity.

Lemon Balm – Reduces stress, improves mood, supports sleep, aids digestion.

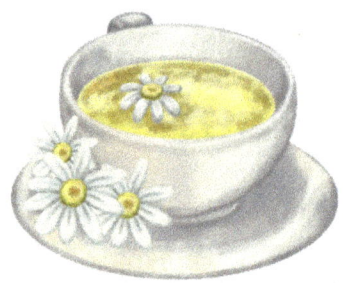
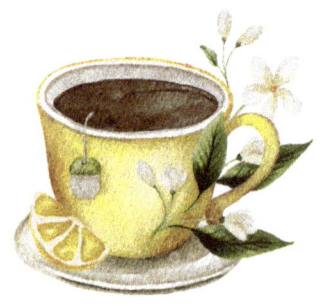

Licorice Root – Soothes sore throat, aids digestion, supports adrenal health, helps with respiratory issues.

Nettle – Anti-inflammatory, supports kidney function, high in minerals, helps with allergies.

Peppermint – Soothes digestion, relieves headaches, freshens breath, reduces bloating.

Rooibos – High in antioxidants, supports heart health, aids digestion, caffeine-free energy booster.

Turmeric – Anti-inflammatory, supports joint health, boosts immunity, aids digestion.

Valerian Root – Promotes deep sleep, reduces anxiety, helps with stress relief.

BLESS YOUR MEALS AND FOOD

When Bill and I moved in together, he suggested we come up with a "Grace" that we can say together before meals. I gifted him the book: **_Graces: Prayers for Everyday Meals and Special Occasions_** by June Cotner, that we still refer to today.

From this book we formulated our own. We look at Lord or G-d as a power for good in the universe, we cannot deny our catholic and jewish roots, so we feel this Non-Denominational prayer prayer covers us all:

Lord, Bless this gathering of our family,
We thank you for the love that unites us.
We thank you, God, for this place in which we live,
For our health, work, food and the freedom that blesses our lives.
Amen.

Bless the earner and bless the cook!

Catholic Grace

Bless us, O Lord, for these, Thy gifts, which we are about to receive from Thy bounty. Through Christ, our Lord. Amen.

Jewish Blessing for the Challah

Baruch ata Adonai Eloheinu Melech ha–olam ha-motz-i lechem min ha'ar-etz.
Blessed is the Oneness that makes us holy and brings forth bread from the earth.
The blessing for the bread covers all the food in your meal.

Buddhist Blessing for Food

Please bless this food that we may take it as a medicine,
With our minds free from attachment and desire.
May it nourish our bodies so that we can work
for the benefit of all sentient beings.

Give Grace to the Elements

Earth, Wind, Fire, Air and Space combine to make this food.
Numberless beings have their lives and laborers that we may eat.
May we be nourished, that we may nourish life.

Give thanks to farmers, growers, cooks

(even if it is yourself).

OTHER BLESSED IDEAS

Make it a priority to sit when you have a meal, or snack, slow down, allow your body the opportunity to accept the nourishment. We tend to over eat if we are not conscious of what we eat. Digestion starts in your mouth with special enzymes, so by chewing slowly it allows for the enzymes to start breaking down the food, making it easier to digest.

The truth is that food is the prayer; health is the blessing.

Try to do nothing else when eating. Just sit and enjoy each bite. If you are eating with others, enjoy their company. No electronics, no TV, no other distractions, just eat, slowly, mindfully and enjoy. Try it, slow down for the health of it, you've come this far, nourish yourself and smile.

"You become what you think about all day long."

~ Ralph Waldo Emerson

AFFIRMATIONS

I'm a firm believer in positive thinking.

According to Buddha, "What you think you become."

What you think about, you bring about.
What you put energy into, energy comes.
Where your focus goes, energy flows.

If it's gratitude and positivity, more things to be grateful for will be.
If it's negative thinking, more negativity could appear.

Try some right now, see how your mood shifts:

I am healthy and strong
I am beautiful
I have everything I want and need
I am grateful for....

Every Day when you wake up, if you **tell yourself it is going to be a great day**, and make it great, no matter the circumstances, you will have a great day.

Even if something bad happens, try to find a silver lining, there is a plan for us and how we embrace this journey can be the difference in a happy life.

At the end of the day when you put your head on your pillow, : **think of all the things that went well that day.** The more goodness you believe in your life, the more goodness comes.

What are you grateful for today?

CACAO CEREMONY

I try to include this practice during the New and Full moon or any time I need a reason to nourish myself and take a few moments to be grateful. Life is cyclical, so honoring the moon cycle helps me sync with nature. So does this ritual. Dating back to Aztec and Mayan times, Cacao is said to help with grounding and improve your connections to body, mind and soul - did I say chocolate?

Not Quite. Chocolate and Cacao are similar in the fact that they both come from the Cacao plant, but Cacao is minimally processed, free from sugar and additives that we find in so many traditional chocolate bars. Cacao holds flavonoids and antioxidants, along with beneficial elements like magnesium, potassium, and selenium, that protect cells from damage caused by free radicals. This may reduce the risk of chronic diseases.

Ceremonial Cacao means there is even less processing (the less processed the better, right?) and typically sourced from ethically based resources.

The idea of Cacao Ceremony is to set intentions and give yourself some mindful moments to bring those intentions to light. Start by melting your Ceremonial Cacao with warm water. The taste is quite bitter but you can blend with a touch of maple syrup or chopped date to sweeten. Expect a delicious frothy warm, spiritual experience. Creating your own ceremony is a great way to slow down and feel life. Smell, sip, journal, you can light a candle, play spiritual music on your own or as a group. At a New Moon, when you want to set new intentions, at Full Moon, when you are embracing that energy, or any time you want to turn inward to reflect on what's going on outward.

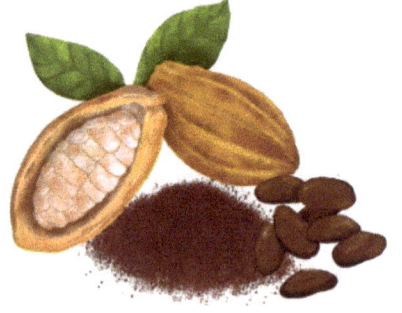 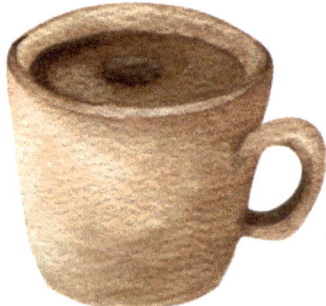 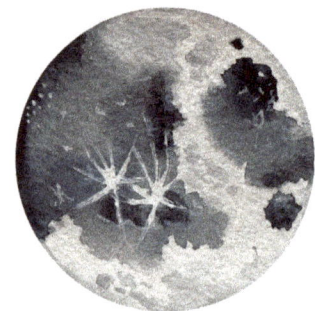

See Reference Guide p.183 for a high quality cacao source.

LOVING KINDNESS MEDITATION

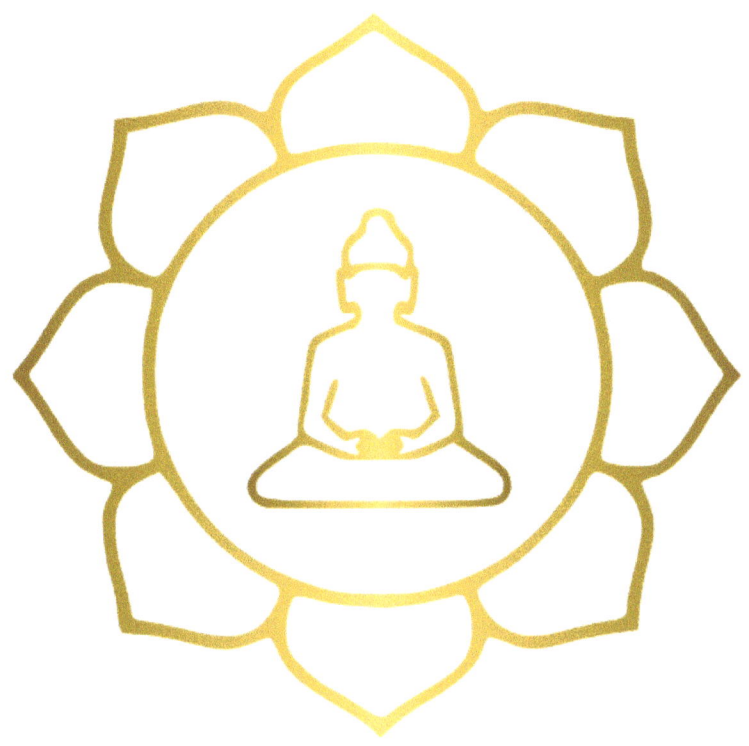

Originating in Buddhism, also known as Metta, Loving Kindness Meditation, was introduced to me by one of my favorite yoga instructors, and dear friend, years ago. I have been studying and using it ever since. You simply send love to yourself, and send it out to the universe. The effects it can have on you and your loved ones are really special. Anywhere, anytime, this string of words and prayers can be used. Say, you miss your kids away at college, send them some good vibes. Or someone cuts you off in traffic, sending some good vibes. I promise it will change your day.

May I be Healthy and strong
May I be Safe
May I be happy
May I be calm and filled with ease
May loving kindness fill my life

Loving-Kindness Meditation

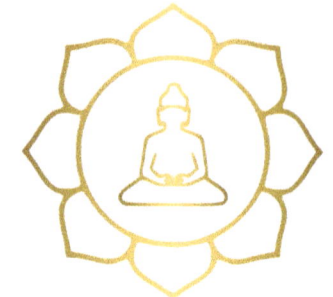

1. Start with by directing the phrases at yourself:
   May I be healthy and strong
   May I be safe
   May I be happy
   May I be calm and filled with ease
   May loving kindness fill my life

2. Next, send this towards someone you love, feel thankful for, or someone who has helped you.
   May You be healthy and strong
   May You be safe
   May You be happy
   May You be calm and filled with ease
   May loving kindness fill your life

3. Now think of someone you feel neutral about—people you neither like nor dislike. This one can be harder than you'd think: (Makes me realize how quick we can be to judge people as either positive or negative in our lives.) examples are: postal worker, grocery clerk, a neighbor that you don't know their name, librarian...
   May You be healthy and strong. May You be happy. May You be calm and filled with ease. May loving kindness fill your life.

4. The next one may be easier: visualizing someone you don't like or who you are having a hard time with. Instead of sending harsh feelings out to the universe - try this - it will fill you up and may have the same effect on them.
   May You be healthy and strong. May You be happy. May You be calm and filled with ease. May loving kindness fill your life.

5. Finally, direct the saying towards everyone universally: **May all beings everywhere be healthy and strong. May all beings everywhere be happy. May all beings everywhere be calm and filled with ease. May all beings everywhere have loving kindness fill their lives.**

THE KITCHEN IS MY TEMPLE

Hint, Hint: This book is a great gift for anyone starting out on their own, here are some ideas and necessities to set up a great healthy kitchen. Even if you're a pro in the kitchen, want to cook more for health reasons, or just intrigued by the idea of mediating while massaging kale, let's explore some ways to build this temple.

Your plate is your altar, what you do to put on it shapes your spirit.

Ways to Meditate while cooking, use your senses: Smell, see, feel all with intention. Smile. Add LOVE to all of your meals. See my recipe for Sauerkraut and you begin to understand.

Good tools you cannot live without:

(Visit www.LandofNutrition.com/kitchen to find links to my favorite products.)

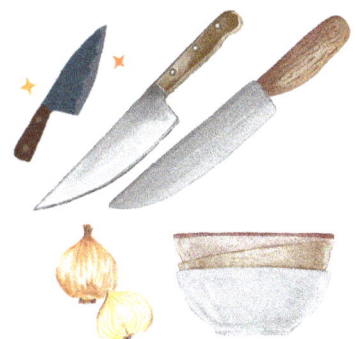

- ✓ Good Knives
- ✓ A chef's most coveted tool. Have a variety of sizes, including a serrated bread knife.
- ✓ Keep them sharp – a dull knife is more dangerous.
- ✓ Wooden Cutting Boards
- ✓ I keep a large one on my counter and use it from sun up (lemon water), to Dinner Prep.
- ✓ Glass storage containers
- ✓ Plastic can contain BPA, a harmful chemical linked to infertility, heart disease, and type 2 diabetes.

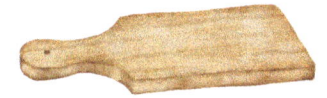

I love the tried and true Brand Pyrex. Many different size and color lids to choose from. I also keep glass jelly jars and pickle jars, give them a good scrub - they make excellent storage containers!

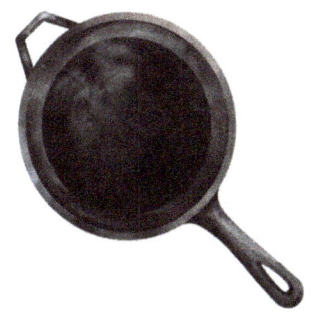

Chemical Safety
Good Quality Pots/Pans:

Choose non-toxic, non aluminum and non teflon (these chemicals have been phased out of manufacturing, but if you still use them or have pans older than 15 years, you may want to consider replacing them).

I love the new ceramic designs from the brand called Our Place, or good stainless steel, which when heated and treated properly can act as a non-stick.

Get a few sizes here, especially the Omelette pan.
Another option that I love is cast iron skillets. Lasting a lifetime with proper care, a true Cast Iron pan adds just that, Iron, to meals, creates great flavor when properly seasoned, heats up evenly and holds the heat easy to clean (absolutely no dish soap or soaking). Steak Au Poivre anyone?

Pots for Boiling Water & Homemade Soups, a few sizes

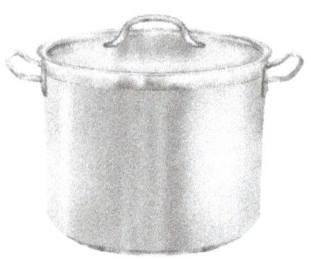

Dutch oven

Perfect for baking sourdough bread

Le Creuset is an investment, but, in my humble opinion, worth it. You can pick them off at garage sales or TJ MAXX store if you know what to look for.

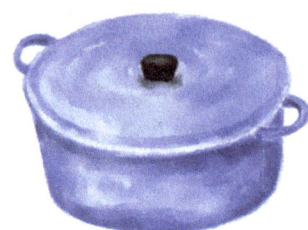

Roasting Pan

Invest in a **good-quality roasting pan** for even cooking, especially good for the comfort meal of whole chicken or turkey dinner.

Plates, Bowls & Platters

Choose items that make you happy and inspire you to cook.

Coffee & Frother Tools

If coffee is your thing, investing in a **good coffee/espresso machine** (I love Breville) can make every morning feel like a vacation.

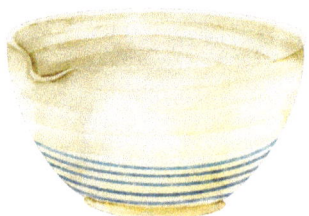

A **countertop frother** is amazing for lattes or matcha — almond milk froths perfectly.

Kitchen Appliances

- ✓ Food processor: Try this beast of a tool - Breville BFP820BAL Sous Chef Peel and Dice 16 Cup Food Processor
- ✓ Toaster Oven: some double as an air fryer
- ✓ High Powered Blender: Vitamix 7500 Blender, Professional-Grade, 64 oz. Low-Profile Container
- ✓ Rice Cooker

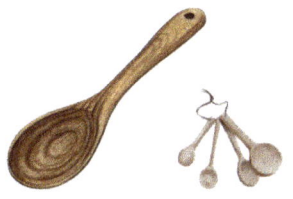

Cooking Utensils

- ✓ Wooden Spoons, Olive wood feels special
- ✓ PBA-free or wooden/silicone spatulas
- ✓ Measuring cups & spoons

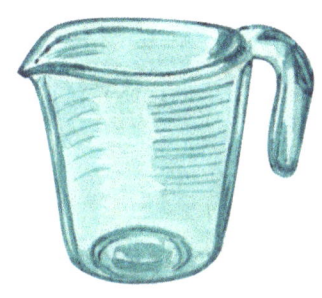

Specialty Tools

- ✓ OXO Good Grips Stainless Steel Salad Spinner, 6.34 Qt.
- ✓ Vegetable peeler
- ✓ This Veggie Chopper was an accidental find (we like to call it a gift from the universe, something that showed up instead of the actual thing I ordered, and I'm in love with it!!), great for easy chopping just be careful, It's very very sharp and have nicked my fingers too many times.
- ✓ Egg slicer (also great for mushrooms)
- ✓ Cheese Grater
- ✓ This is a great scrubber for your "stuck on" cooking needs, made from peach pits, eco friendly and really works - Looks like Spagetti Scrubber
- ✓ A stainless steel "soap" - great for removing garlic and fish smells from your hands
- ✓ Pineapple slicer that takes out the core (keep it for smoothies), there's a story that includes blood that lead to this purchase too.
- ✓ Countertop Compost bucket (great for the environment, bonus if you use it in your garden).

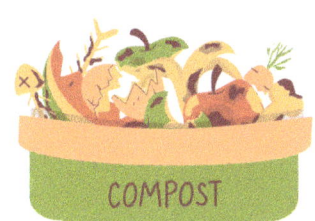

Organizational Tools

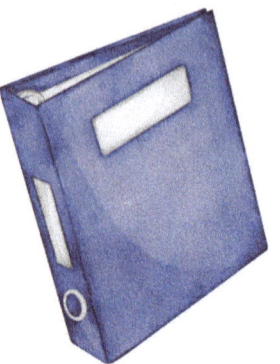

- ✓ Notepad nearby for ideas and grocery lists
- ✓ 3-Ring Binder with page protectors for recipes — keep only the ones you love and use.
- ✓ Cookbook holder - so you can prop this up all pretty.
- ✓ Cooking becomes second nature when you have the right tools.

Keep what you love, let go of clutter, and enjoy your time in the kitchen.

In Part 2 of *Food is My Religion*, you will find an array of everyday and special occasion meals, side dishes and healthy desserts that I whip up regularly in my own temple - my kitchen.

Visit *www.LandofNutrition.com/kitchen* to find links to my favorite products.

We may receive a portion of sales if you purchase a product through these links. Thank you for your consideration when shopping through my links.

NOTES:

THE GOLDEN RULE

When Bill and I were about to marry, someone told us that having two religions would never work. 25 years later, we have a thriving family based in love and kindness (with a love for good food). With each of our three children is a beautiful spirituality that makes a parent proud.

What do Religions have in common?

Dating back to ancient Egyptian and Greek times, thousands of years ago, common themes of ethical and moral behavior have been found, guiding followers to treat each other with kindness, compassion and respect.

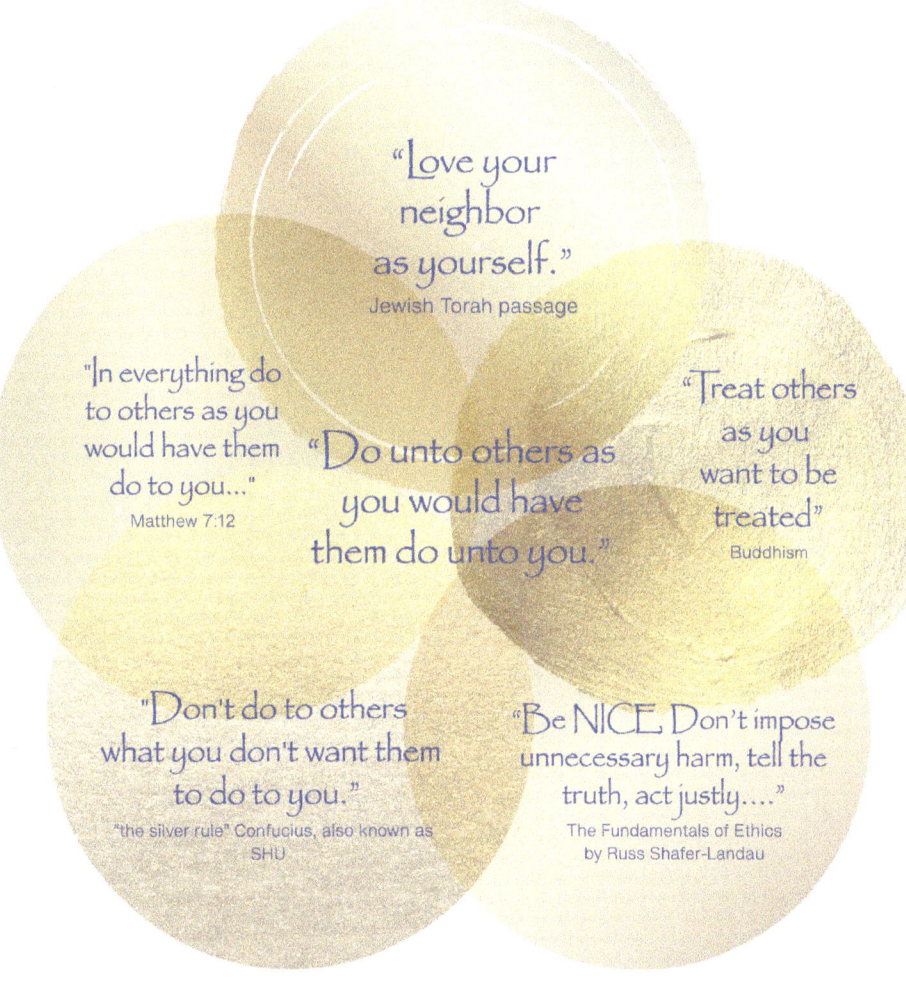

GETTING TO THE ROOT OF WHAT NOURISHES YOU

You need to know yourself to live a happy and fulfilled life and why not make it the happiest and healthiest you can. Fill your cup of life first and the love you have within will spill over to those around you. Eat like you love yourself, because you are worth it.

It's always a good idea to journal to get some insight into what you believe in.
What's your whole story?
Are you happy?
Do you know what makes you happy?
Because if you don't know what makes you happy, how could you possibly make others happy?
Root deep with me in health and wellness, let's find your meaning of life.
Answering some of these questions can help you slow down, reflect inward, and take the time for yourself.
You deserve it.
And know that the joy is in the journey, there's no end.

NOTES:

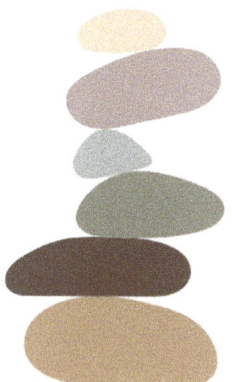
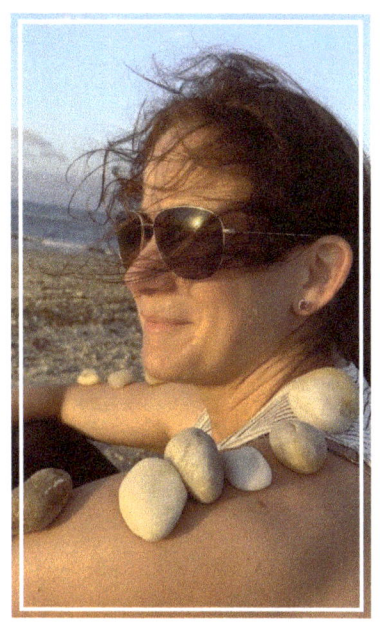

Life is a balancing act

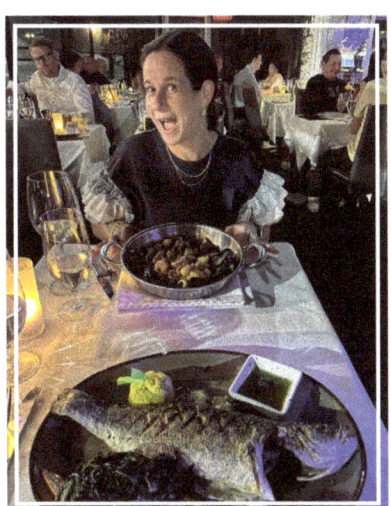
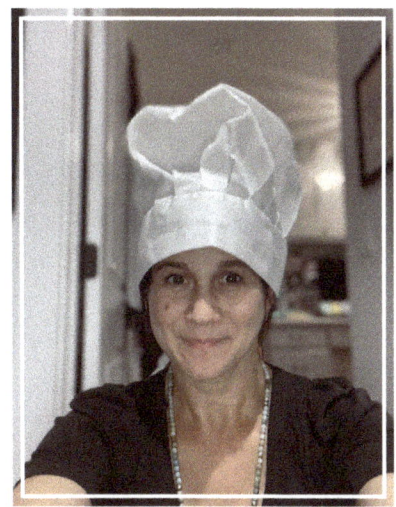
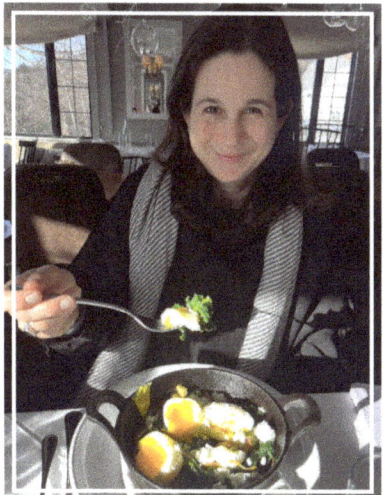

What makes you happy?

MEAL PLANNING

Meal Plan like there is a tomorrow and the next day and the next day.

Adulting is hard, like having to decide what's for dinner. Every. Single. Day.

When we meal plan and prepare, we are setting ourselves up for successful health-full meals, which is the end goal, right?

What's for dinner? The million dollar question we dread. Changing our mindsets here.

Getting to the kitchen early, 10-15 minutes more of relaxed prep can make all the difference. So make yourself a mocktail and start the process of nurturing with simple, delicious, healthy meals.

See Part 2 for tried and true recipes to get you through.

You can have a process that each day of the week assigns a type of meal.

Here's an easy guide for you to no-brainer dinners, based on the day of the week - make it your own and know that YES, every day can be Taco Day. And Breakfast for dinner is a thing.

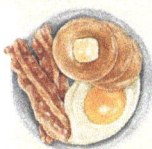
Meatless Monday
had its moment, Breakfast for dinner is always a hit: Eggs, Bacon, Pancakes, Waffles, add some fruit for bonus points. Keep the meatless with a delicious bean or lentil soup loaded up with kale or swiss chard.

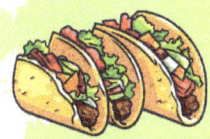
Taco Tuesday
Burrito, tortilla pizzas, enchiladas, they are all the same ingredients, just prepared in different ways.

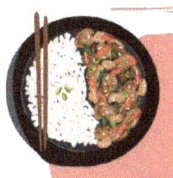
International Wednesday
Italian Meatballs, Greek falafel, Asian pork wraps - Prepare rice and add chicken, ground pork or your choice of protein. Fried Rice, add green, sautéed kale or spinach, heat rice and crack an egg in the middle and whisk away until the egg is incorporated into the rice, add peas or any veggie you like.

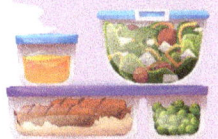
Leftover Thursday
Thursday is for leftovers, Mix it up, rice and beans, mediterranean platter with tzatziki, hummus, pitas, chickpea salad, or TACO NIGHT again!

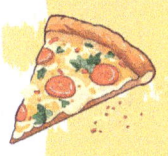
Pizza Friday
It's Pizza Night, remember the salad and protein.

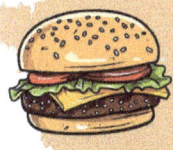
Go-with-the-flow Saturday
Leave Saturday for going with the flow, going out to dinner or ordering in. Try Hamburgers, Hot Dogs, Salad (You should have the time to make a beautiful salad, remember to meditate while chopping veggies).

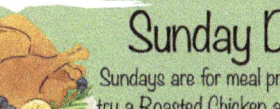
Sunday Dinner/Family Night
Sundays are for meal prep and maybe a Sunday Night dinner roast, order sushi, try a Roasted Chicken and/or Grill Some steak and potatoes, caramelized onion and the mushrooms you got from the farmers market over the weekend.

Use the food day guides (on the next pages) for meal planning ideas: oh it's national hotdog day let's have a hotdog (make sure it is grass fed organic beef)! Sauerkraut is so good for you - lop it on (try my homemade sauerkraut recipe, or make sure you read the label to get the real deal) Is a hot dog a sandwich? Is cereal a soup?

It's National Lasagna Day, let's have lasagna! Fill it with veggies and add a salad.

Purposely not including a Meal Plan here - I want to give you the power to create what you like.

And remember: Meals don't have to be on a plate, a BOWL is a great idea – load up on veggies, add some protein, grains, a little healthy fat and you are good to go!

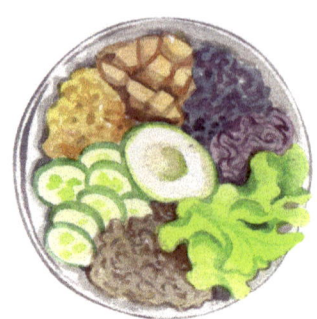

Have a Prep Fest. Have a flexible weekly meal prep plan:
Take a few hours when you can, most choose a few hours on a Sunday, or pick a day that works for you, set aside 2-3 hours to make meals easy all week. Double recipes, use leftovers for lunch, it's called batch cooking, you got this.

- ✓ Chop & store veggies (carrots, cruciferous veggies, leafy greens).
- ✓ Cook a batch of quinoa or brown rice.
- ✓ Roast sweet potatoes (store them in the fridge for easy meals).
- ✓ Prepare a protein (bake salmon, ground beef or chicken).
- ✓ Make raw carrot salad (store it in an airtight container in the refrigerator for daily servings).
- ✓ Boil eggs (great for snacks).
- ✓ Prep a smoothie mix (freeze berries, spinach, and chia seeds in a bag for easy blender prep).

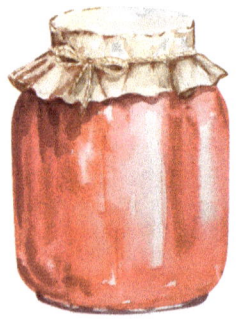
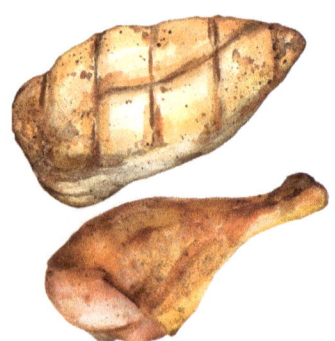
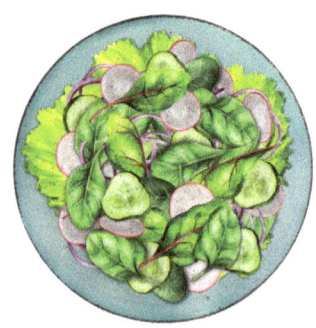

CELEBRATE FOOD EVERYDAY

FOOD IS MY RELIGION FOOD HOLIDAYS

There's a reason to celebrate food everyday! I've combed the web and culminated my findings, going to admit, most are sugar laden and not the best health choices, like National Cheese Doodle Day, so here is the **Food is My Religion** healthy food of the day for each day of the year.

Some of them are actual National or International "holidays," as noted with a "*".
If there is an "^" sign, look for the recipe with that ingredient in Part 2 of this book!
If you are meal planning and get stuck, take a look!
If you have a favorite food and there's a day - then celebrate!
If you miss a day, no worries, celebrate today!

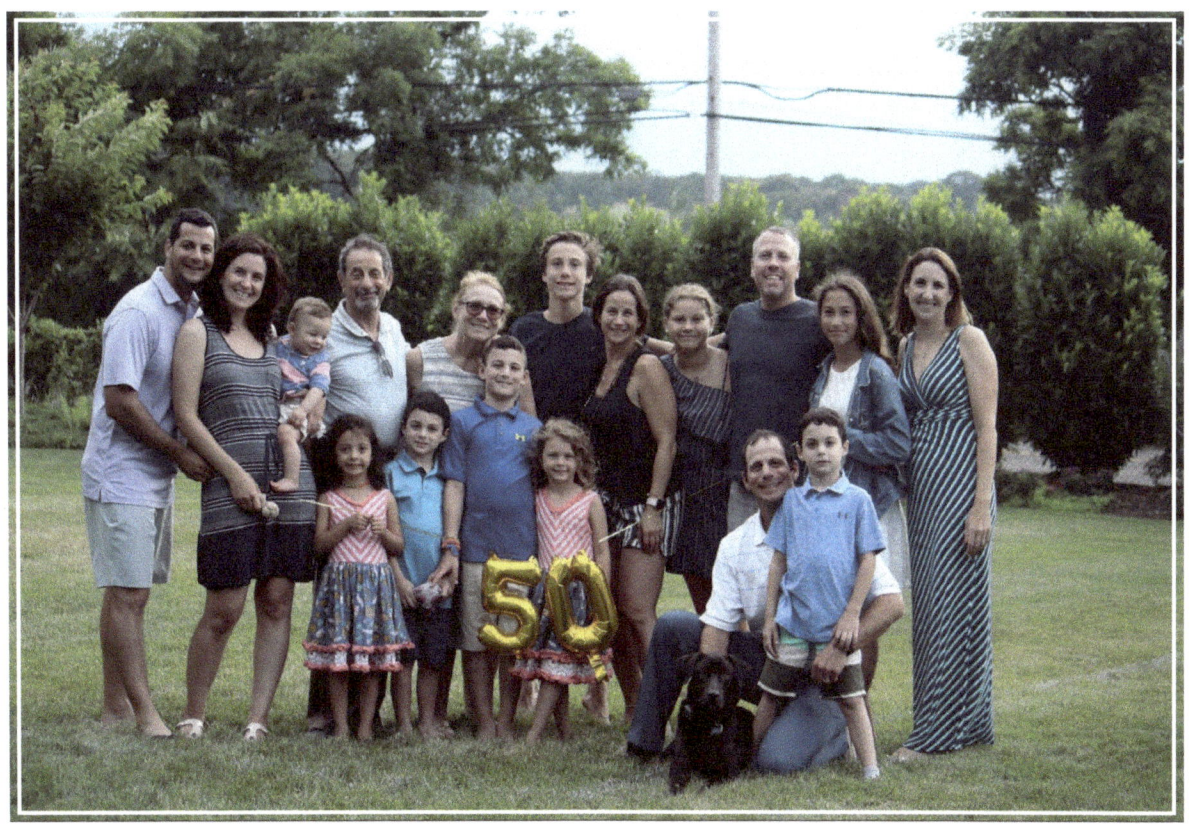

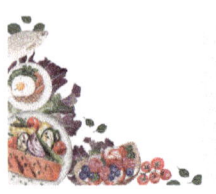

365 Day
Food Is My Religion Healthy Food Calendar

January (Winter Wellness)

1. Pomegranate Seed Day for good luck into the new year
2. National Buffet Day*
3. National Chocolate Covered Cherry Day* - Have a Black forest smoothie
4. National Spaghetti Day* (bonus: make it zoodles)
5. Grass Fed Steak Day
6. National Bean Day*
7. Chicken Cutlet Day^
8. Broccoli Day
9. Dried Apricot Day*
10. Almond Day
11. National Milk Day*
12. Cauliflower Day^
13. Chia Seed Day^
14. Winter Squash Day^
15. Sweet Potato Day
16. International Hot and Spicy Day*
17. Olive Oil Day^
18. National Gourmet Coffee Day*
19. National Popcorn Day*
20. Bell Pepper Day
21. Granola Bar Day*
22. Flaxseed Day^
23. Organic Tofu Day
24. Sauerkraut Day ^
25. Sticky Rice Bowl Day
26. National Green Juice Day*
27. Caramelized Onions Day^
28. National Blueberry Pancake Day* (Breakfast for Dinner, anyone?)
29. Oats Day^
30. National Croissant Day* (One of my Favorite things on earth), also National Brussel Sprouts Day*
31. National Hot Chocolate Day* (let's make our own)

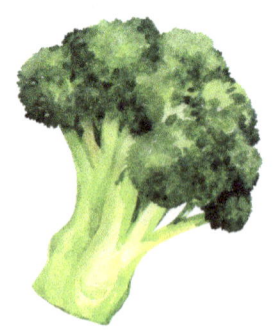

February (Heart Healthy Choices)

1. National Dark Chocolate Day*
2. National Crepe Day*
3. Cabbage Day^
4. National Homemade Soup Day*
5. Caramelized Onions Day^
6. National use Chop Sticks Day*
7. Raspberries Day^
8. National Potato Day*
9. National Pizza Day*
10. Hummus Day
11. Pumpkin Seeds Day^
12. Farro Day
13. Greek Salad Day
14. Valentine's Day Beets Day
15. Lentil Soup Day
16. National Almond Day*
17. National Cabbage Day*^
18. Artichoke Day
19. Coconut Oil Day^
20. National Muffin Day*^
21. Mango Day^
22. Sweet Potato Day^
23. National Banana Bread Day*^
24. Carrot Day^
25. National Chocolate Covered Nuts Day*
26. National Pistachio Day*
27. National Strawberry Day*^
28. Olive You Day

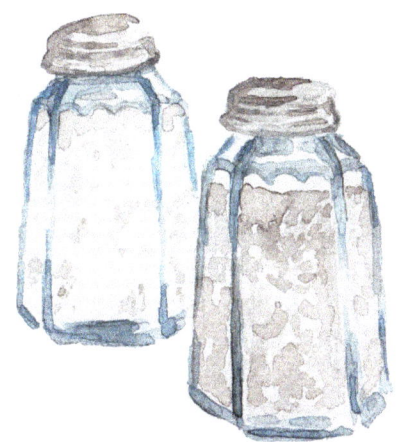
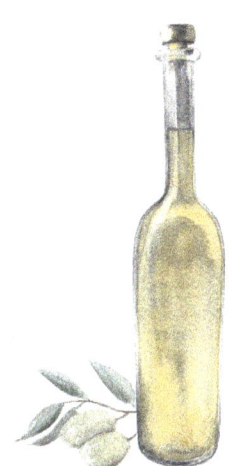

March (Spring Ahead)

1. National Fruit Compote Day*
2. Carrot Cake Day
3. Almond Butter Day^
4. National Pancakes Day*
5. Grapes Day
6. National Frozen Fruit Day*^
7. Hemp Seed Day
8. Cashew Day
9. National Crabmeat Day*
10. Blackberry Day
11. Chicken Thigh Day
12. Seaweed Day
13. Herbal Tea Day^
14. Pi(e) Day 3.14.........
15. Peas Day
16. National Artichoke Day*
17. St Patrick's Day / Cabbage Day / Irish Soda Bread Day^
18. Papaya Day
19. Turmeric Rice Day^
20. National Sauerkraut Day*^
21. Pecans Day
22. Kimchi Day
23. National Chips & Dip Day*
24. Honeydew Day
25. Breakfast for Dinner National Waffle Day*
26. Collard Greens Day
27. National Paella Day*
28. Cucumber Salad Day
29. Tuna Day
30. Soba Noodles Day
31. Cacao Day^

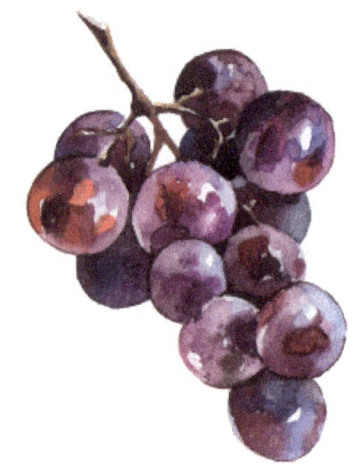

April (Spring Bounty)

1. National Sourdough Day*^
2. National PB&J Day*
3. National Chocolate Mousse Day*
4. Mustard Greens Day
5. Dandelion day – Dandelions are edible Day
6. French Radish Day*
7. Coconut Cream Day
8. Kale Chips Day
9. Duck Eggs Day
10. Leg of Lamb Day
11. Zucchini Noodles Day
12. Goji Berry Day
13. Chicken Salad Day
14. Blood Orange Day
15. National Banana Day*^
16. Falafel & Tzatziki Day^
17. Black Beans Day^
18. Caramelized Onion Day^
19. Garlic Cloves Day^
20. Wild Rice Day
21. Plantains Day^
22. Carrot Ginger Dressing Day^
23. Skirt Steak & Chimichurri Day^
24. Endive Day
25. Almond Milk Day
26. National Zucchini Bread Day*
27. Dutch Pancake Day
28. Chives Day^
29. Chia Seed Pudding Day
30. Dried Fruit Day

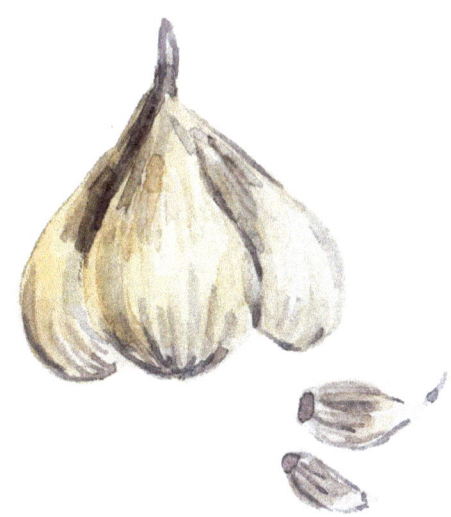

CELEBRATE FOOD EVERYDAY

May (Fresh Selections)

1. National Salad Day*^
2. National Matcha Day*
3. Quinoa Bowl Day
4. Mango Salsa Day^
5. TACO Day/Cinco de Mayo
6. NO DIET DAY
7. Green Beans Day^
8. Lemon Day
9. National Shrimp Day*
10. Sweet Basil Day
11. Apricot Jam Day
12. Almond Flour Day
13. National Hummus Day*
14. Cucumber Lemon Spa Day^
15. Great Northern White Beans Day^
16. National BBQ Day*^
17. Coconut Day^
18. Honey Day^
19. Nori Day
20. World Bee Day*
21. International Tea Day*^
22. Radish Day
23. Egg Salad Day
24. Roasted Chickpeas Day
25. Sweet Pepper Day
26. Dill Day
27. Cherries Jubilee Day
28. National Burger Day*
29. Boston Bibb Lettuce Day^
30. International Day of Potato*^
31. Coconut Macaroons Day^

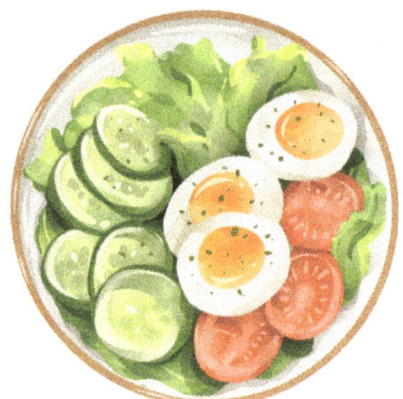
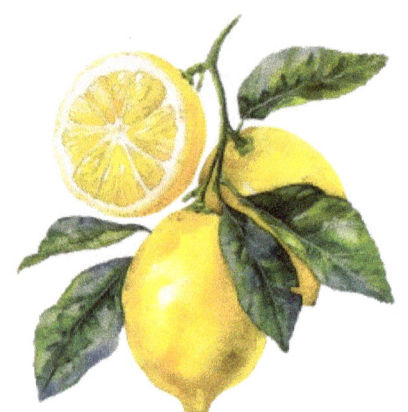

June (Farmer's Market Feasts)

1. Watermelon Day
2. Fennel Salad Day
3. National Egg Day*
4. National Cheese Day*
5. Make a Berry Board Day^
6. Bok Choy Day
7. Farro Salad Day
8. Banana Day^
9. Grilled Shrimp Day
10. National Iced Tea Day
11. Cucumber Mint Salad Day
12. National Falafel, Mediterranean Meatballs and Tzatziki Day*^
13. French Radish Day
14. Tahini Day^
15. National Lobster Day*
16. Chamomile Day^
17. National "Eat Your Vegetables Day"*^
18. International Sushi Day*
19. Parmesan is a Protein Day
20. Arugula Pesto Pasta Day
21. National Smoothie Day*
22. Summer Squash Day
23. Fennel Day
24. Coconut Rice Day
25. Balsamic Vinegar Day
26. Greens Galore Day
27. Tofu Lettuce Wraps Day
28. Citrus Celebration Day
29. Sushi Day
30. Lemon Basil Chicken Day

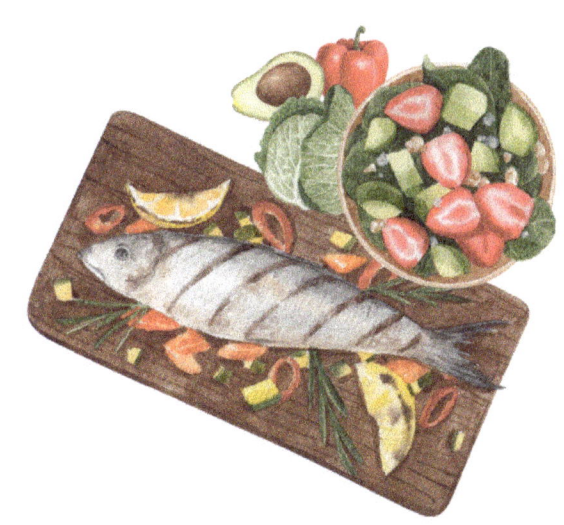

July (Fresh Selections)

1. International Chicken Wing Day*
2. Fajita Day
3. National "Eat Beans" Day*
4. Grass Fed Beef Hot Dog Day
5. Tomato Basil Bruschetta Day
6. Cucumber Dill Salad Day
7. World Chocolate Day*^
8. Watermelon Feta Salad Day
9. Cilantro Lime Chicken Day
10. National Pick Blueberries Day*
11. National Blueberry Muffin Day
12. Grilled Artichokes Day
13. National French Fry Day*^
14. Roasted Red Pepper Day
15. Cherries Day
16. Spicy Black Bean Dip Day
17. Chilled Gazpacho Day
18. Sweet Potato Fries Day
19. Garlic Butter Shrimp Day
20. National Ice Cream Day*
21. Granola Day^
22. Herb-Crusted Salmon Day
23. National Chocolate & Peanut Butter Day*
24. Lemon Garlic Hummus Day
25. Heirloom Tomato Day
26. Green Beans Day^
27. Grilled Pineapple Day
28. Zucchini Fritters Day
29. National Chicken Wing Day*
30. Spinach Feta Stuffed Chicken Day
31. National Avocado Day*

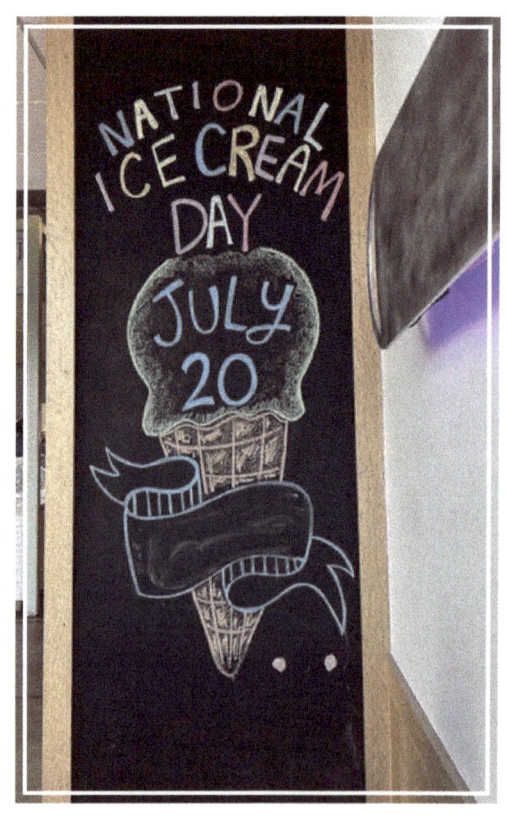

August (Summer Sessions)

1. Vegetable Stir-fry Day
2. Quinoa Fried Rice Day
3. National Watermelon Day*
4. Chicken Shawarma Day
5. National Oyster Day*
6. Raspberry Vinaigrette Day^
7. Summer Salad Day^
8. National Zucchini Day*
9. Roasted Chickpea Salad Day
10. Lemon Herb Grilled Fish Day
11. Peaches Day
12. Carrot Ginger Soup Day
13. Stuffed Bell Peppers Day
14. Zucchini Muffin Day^
15. Gazpacho Day^
16. National Honey Bee (use the honey) Day*^
17. Eggplant Parmesan Day
18. Honey Garlic Chicken Day
19. Summer Vegetable Ratatouille Day
20. Corn and Avocado Salsa Day
21. Coconut Lime Rice Day
22. National Eat a Peach Day*
23. Grilled Chicken Caesar Salad Day^
24. Zucchini & Ground Turkey Boats Day
25. Fresh Basil Lemonade Day
26. Tomato Basil Soup Day
27. National Burger Day*
28. Baba Ganoush Day
29. Grilled Vegetable Sandwich Day
30. International Bacon Day* (just make sure it's NO Nitrate/Nitrites)
31. National Eat Outside Day*

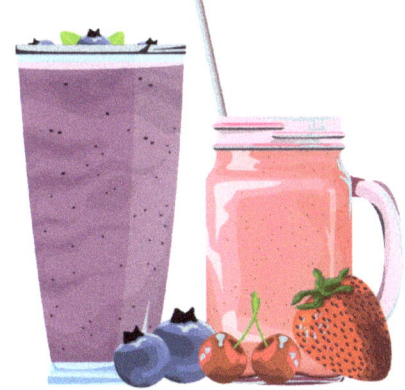
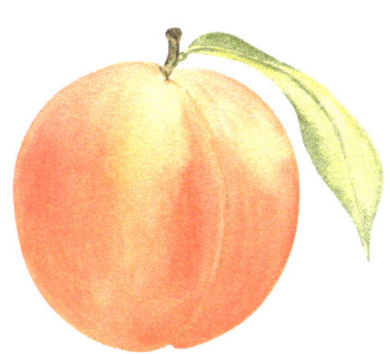

CELEBRATE FOOD EVERYDAY

September (Beat the Heat)

1. National Gyro Day*
2. National "Eat Your Veggies" Day*^
3. Pickled Onion Day^
4. Grilled Chicken Fajitas Day
5. Honeycrisp Apple Day
6. Honey Mustard Brussels Sprouts Day
7. National Acorn Squash Day*
8. Quinoa & Black Bean with Fried Egg Bowl Day
9. Chicken Noodle Soup Day
10. Apple Cider Vinegar Day
11. Basil Pesto and Caprese Salad Day
12. Shrimp Taco Day
13. Kale & Quinoa Salad Day
14. TNT Fish Taco Day^
15. Sweet Potato Toasts Day
16. Scrambled Eggs Day
17. National Guacamole Day*
18. Maple Roasted Carrots Day
19. Grilled Chicken Day
20. Pumpkin Spice Smoothie Day
21. Cantaloupe Day
22. Lemon Garlic Roasted Chicken Day
23. Roasted Cauliflower Day
24. Apple Crisp Day
25. Apple Walnut Salad Day
26. Buckwheat Pancakes Day
27. National Chocolate Milk Day*
28. Chicken and Broccoli Stir-fry Day
29. National Coffee Day*
30. Pumpkin Pancakes Day

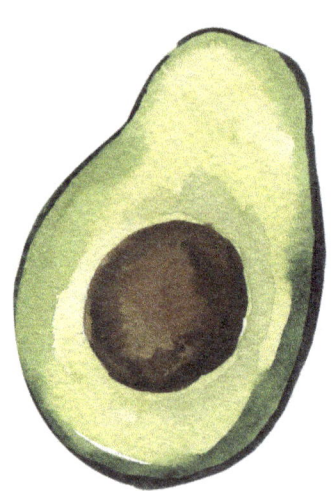

October (Autumn Harvest)

1. World Vegetarian Day* and National Kale Day* (first Wednesday of October)
2. Cape Cod Cod Day^
3. Ground Turkey Burger Day
4. Butternut Squash Day
5. Spicy Chickpea Stew Day
6. Pumpkin Soup Day
7. National Taco Day*
8. Stuffed Bell Peppers Day
9. Carrot Hummus Day
10. Chocolate AVO Mousse Day
11. Roasted Beets Day
12. Sweet Potato Mash Day
13. Sautéed Garlic Spinach Day
14. Chicken Vegetable Stir-fry Day
15. National Mushroom Day* - Try Grilled Portobello Mushrooms
16. WORLD FOOD DAY and National Oatmeal Day*
17. Maple Roasted Brussels Sprouts Day
18. Pumpkin Seed Granola Day
19. Apples & Cinnamon Day
20. Chicken Tortilla Soup Day
21. National Apple Day*
22. National Nut Day*
23. Roasted Vegetable Day
24. Lemon Garlic Broccoli Day
25. Black Bean and Corn Salad Day
26. Pumpkin Spice Latte
27. National Potato Day*
28. National Chocolate Day*
29. Banana Pancake Day
30. Pear Crisp Day
31. Halloween Chili Day

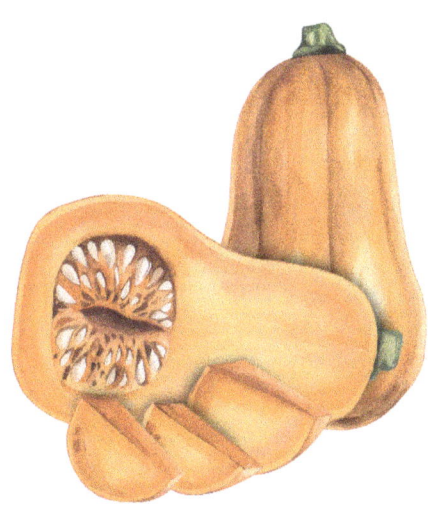

November (Holiday Nutrition)

1. World VEGAN Day and National Cinnamon Day*^
2. Broccoli Potato Soup Day
3. National Sandwich Day*
4. National Eating Healthy Day*
5. Cranberry Sauce Day
6. National Nacho Day*
7. Maple Glazed Carrots Day
8. Cauliflower Day^
9. Pomegranate Salad Day
10. Ceviche Day^
11. Roasted Chicken Thighs Day^
12. Brussels Sprouts with Bacon Day
13. Dates Day^
14. National Pickle Day*
15. Red Lentil Soup Day
16. Homemade Bread Day*
17. Pumpkin Butter Spread Day
18. Cauliflower Tacos Day
19. Roasted Root Vegetables Day
20. Ground Pork Lettuce Wraps Day
21. National Cranberry Day*
22. National Cashew Day*
23. Turkey Sandwich Day
24. Leftover Turkey Soup Day
25. Sweet Potato and Kale Hash Day
26. Cranberry Almond Energy Bites Day
27. Maple Latte Day
28. Vegetable Frittata Day^
29. Stuffed Mushrooms Day
30. Orange and Fennel Salad Day

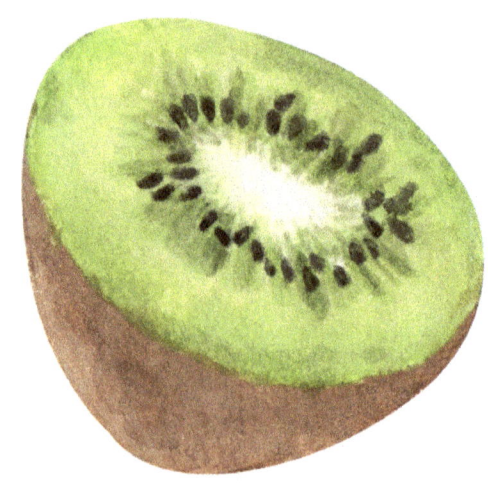

December (Winter Superfoods)

1. Butternut Squash Soup Day^
2. Roasted Chestnuts Day
3. Kiwi Day
4. Holiday Cookie Day^
5. National Comfort Food Day*^
6. Gingerbread Day
7. Spinach and Mushroom Quiche Day
8. Peppermint Hot Chocolate with Almond Milk Day
9. Roasted Delicata Squash Harvest Bowl Day
10. Figgy Pudding Day
11. Horchata Chia Pudding Day
12. Sweet Potato Gnocchi Day
13. National Cocoa Day*
14. Holiday Brisket Day^
15. Potato Latke Day^
16. National Chocolate Covered ANYTHING Day*
17. National Maple Syrup Day*
18. Charcuterie Board Day
19. Winter Vegetable Soup Day
20. Peppermint Smoothie Day
21. National Hamburger Day*
22. Roasted Beets Day
23. Lasagna Day
24. Christmas Eve Feast Day
25. Christmas Roast Day^
26. Turkey and Vegetable Stir-fry Day
27. Leftover Feast Day
28. Kale & Sausage Day
29. New Year's Eve Appetizers Day
30. Black Eyed Peas for Good Luck Day
31. National Champagne Day* Cheers to Health

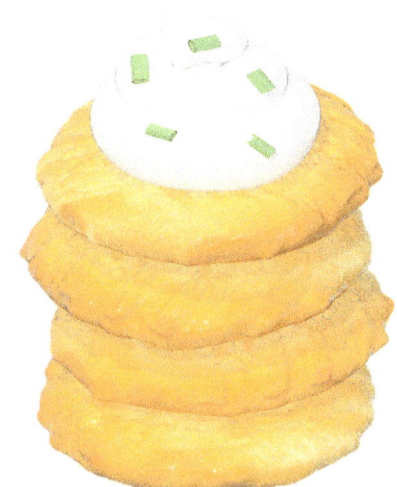

CELEBRATE FOOD EVERYDAY

WRAPPING IT UP WITH GRATITUDE

Institute for Integrative Nutrition opened my eyes to many health topics and theories, with highly regarded health professional instructors. I am so grateful for the program and all I've learned and digested. Learning healthy habits that go way beyond our plate is at the core. The truth is, there is no one path for all. We're all different and need to find what is best for each of us. There's so much (too much) information out there, pay attention to your specific needs, situations and know that things change and will change for different circumstances. There are some overlapping ideals that are important for the health of everyone though–things we can all benefit from: Quality sleep, hydration and nutrition from unprocessed, whole foods, staying away from harmful ingredients.

Food is a tool for Health - It's your choices that will make a difference in your Health. Just think: HEALTHY = HEAL THY - you can heal yourself with your food choices. You can prevent disease with this awareness.

Take a moment to thank yourself, be grateful for your beautiful bodies, and take time to think about your health and what's attributing to it and what may be taking away from it. What are you digesting in terms of spirituality, relationships, exercise, career, what you consume on your plate, your social media, the people you surround yourself with? Please know that whoever, wherever you are, there is someone routing for you, cheering you on to be the best you can be – never stop improving.

> *I believe in you and the power to change your health and mindset for the better.*

I am so grateful for you, dear reader, for making it to the end of this book. Thank you for being here. Thank you for holding this book, my heart, in your hands and on your book shelves.

Stay tuned for Part 2, where I share every day and holiday recipes from my Temple to yours.
Be Well,

xoxo Lara

The 10 Commandments of Food Is My Religion

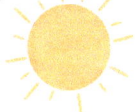 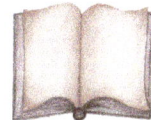 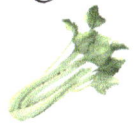 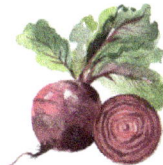

1. Choose Whole Foods.
Eat close to nature — local, seasonal, and high quality whenever you can. Build balance with vegetables, fruits, proteins, healthy fats, whole grains, and plenty of hydration.

2. Read Labels Carefully. Avoid the Naughty List ingredients.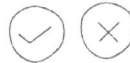
Know what's going into your body. Skip ingredients you don't recognize or wouldn't cook with yourself.

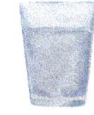

3. Eat with Intention. Bless this Meal.
Slow down. Sit, breathe, and give your full attention to your meal. Gratitude and presence make food more nourishing.

4. Move Daily.
Keep your body flowing — walk, stretch, dance, smile. Repeat often, and make movement part of everyday life.

5. Be Smart About Sugar.
Sugar has its place, but let it be the exception, not the rule. Find healthier swaps and savor treats mindfully.

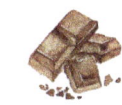

6. Create Meaningful Rituals.
Step outside in the morning light, brew your coffee or tea with intention, and let small daily practices set the tone for your day.

7. Cook at Home. The Kitchen is My Temple.
The kitchen is where real nourishment begins. Cooking for yourself (and others) is one of the most powerful acts of care.

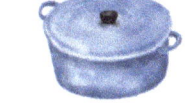

8. Practice the Golden Rule. Treat people how you want to be treated (this includes yourself). Treat your body, your food, and those you share meals with - with the utmost respect.

9. Celebrate Food Every Day.
Every snack, meal, and gathering is a chance to enjoy and appreciate. Celebrate both the simple and the special.

10. Remember Food is Health. And Health is Wealth.
What you eat shapes your health, your energy, and your joy. Choose food that supports the life you want to live.

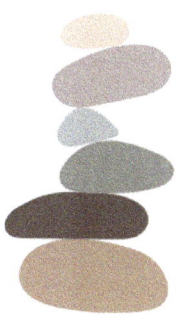

NOTES:

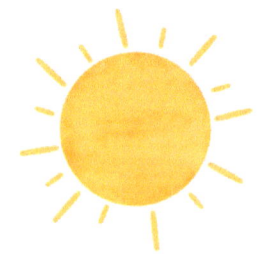

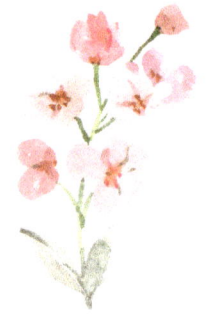

grateful

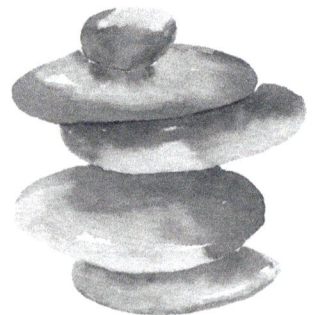

I love food — the nourishment it gives, the stories it carries, the laughter around a shared table, the quiet comfort of a meal alone. Food is my ritual, my joy, my religion.

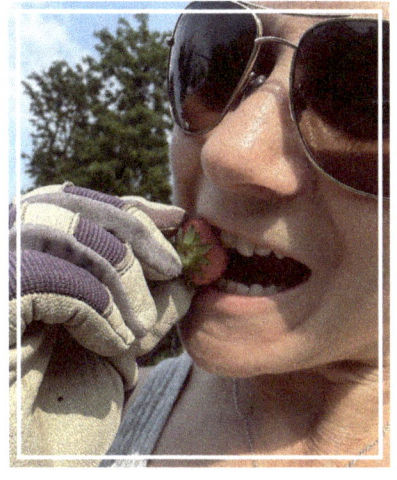
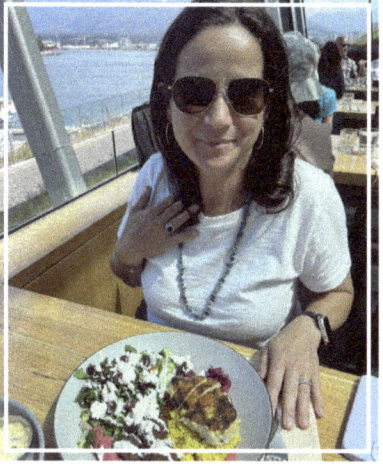
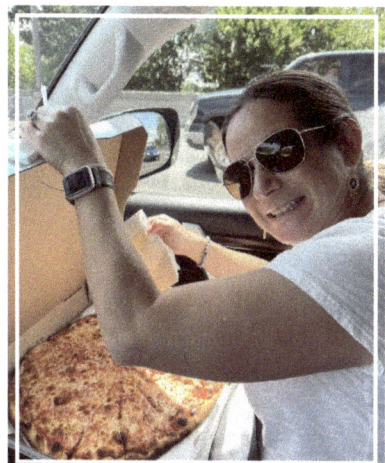
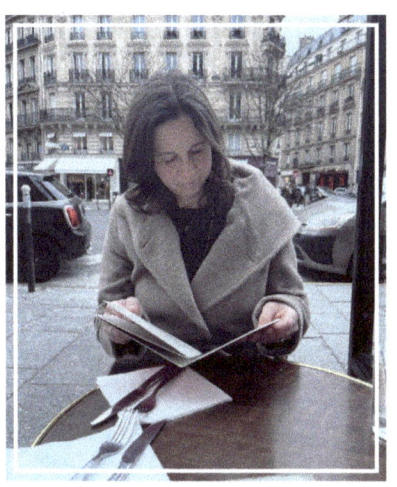
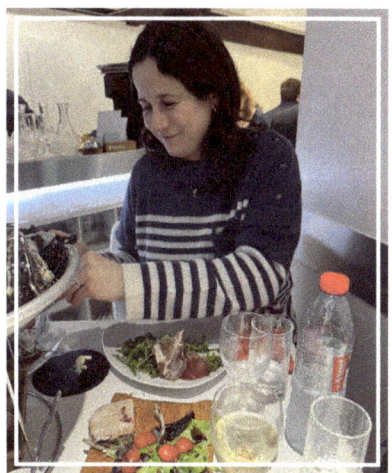
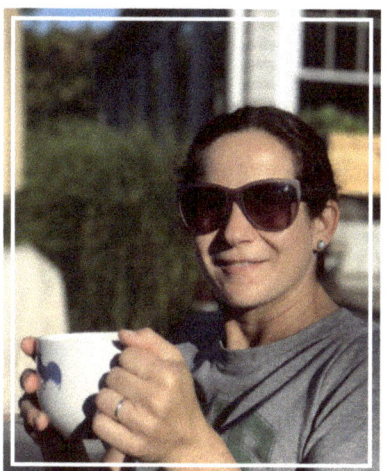
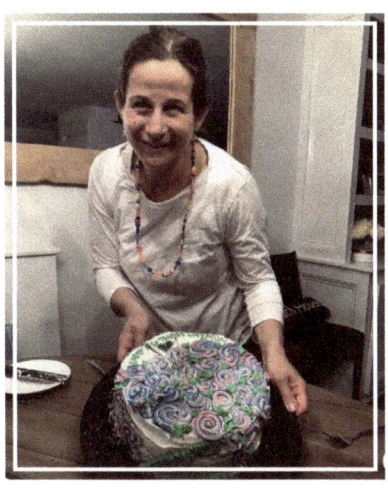
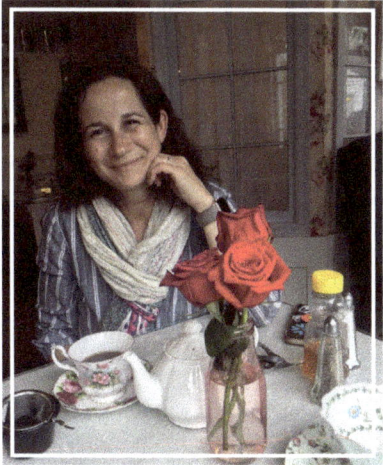
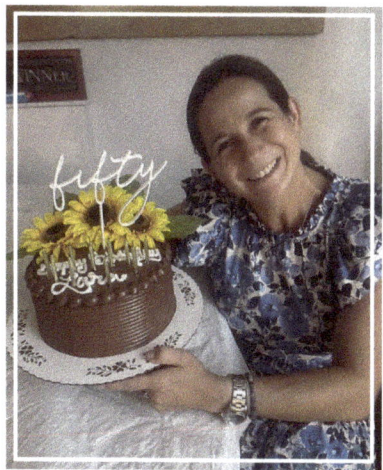

Food is My Religion

Part 2 Recipes

Selfishly, I have organized my go-to recipes in one spot. I have little pieces of paper, post-it notes (one of my favorite inventions), index cards, print outs and magazine cut outs all over the place. A binder with plastic sleeves is an amazing way to corral recipes, by the way, but writing this book has been fun. I also like to amend recipes with what I have in stock, what's in my pantry and sub a healthier ingredient in here and there.

The way I cook is simple, few ingredients and wing it. You can teach yourself to love cooking simple healthy meals and worship food, as it is a direct link to your health.

I'm offering some guidance here and a peek into the Land of Nutrition Kitchen, my Temple.

The recipes on the following pages are good for you and good for celebrating all occasions. These are recipes for all days and holidays.

I encourage you to make every day a holiday and make these your own, mix and match salads, main meals and sides.

Here are some of my favorites.
Enjoy!

xoxo Lara

Key
T=Tablespoon (Big T)
t=teaspoon (little t)
EVOO = Extra Virgin Olive Oil
GF = Gluten Free

Salads, Dressings, Sauces and Dips

LAND OF NUTRITION EVERYDAY HOMEMADE SALAD DRESSING

(Never buy store-bought dressing again). Look for EVOO in a glass container bottled from a single origin and cold pressed. Extra Virgin Olive Oil (EVOO) is a healthy fat, best consumed unheated, promotes heart health and reduces inflammation. The polyphenols in EVOO act like prebiotics, feeding beneficial gut bacteria and supporting a healthy microbiome.

INGREDIENTS:

- ✓ 1/4 cup Good Extra Virgin Olive Oil
- ✓ 1/4 cup White Balsamic Vinegar (Red Wine Vinegar or Fresh Squeezed Lemon Juice work great too)
- ✓ 1-2 tsp Dijon mustard
- ✓ Pinch of Sea Salt & Pepper

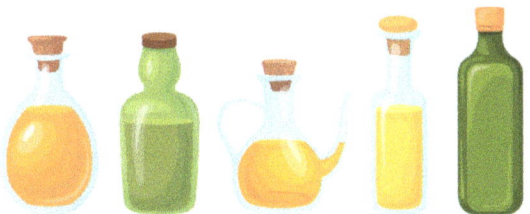

Put all in a Salad Dressing Jar and shake
Enjoy!
Keep on countertop for up to a week

BABY GREENS SALAD

Organic Delicate Baby Greens are tender young leaves bursting with vitamins, minerals, and antioxidants—an easy daily devotion to fresh, living nourishment (This is truly all you need for this simple salad, add thinly sliced red onion, shaved carrots, or whatever veggies you have on hand that you love)!

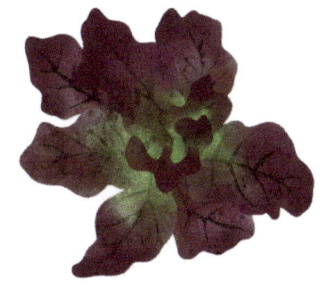

Serve as a side dish for any meal, especially yummy with an omelet or frittata.

CONCORD SALAD

We recreated this one from a beautiful farm to table restaurant experience. Use Lettuce Gem Greens, Crispy Baby Green Leaf, the brand "Gotham Greens" has an awesome bag of "Ugly Greens," the key is to soak them in cold water to freshen them up, drain them and give them a spin in a salad spinner.

I'M PURPOSELY LEAVING OFF MEASUREMENTS, YOU DO YOU:

- ✓ Lettuce
- ✓ Apple Sliced Thin - any apple variety will work here
- ✓ Avocado cubed
- ✓ Sunflower seeds
- ✓ Red onion sliced thin
- ✓ Crumbled goat cheese
- ✓ Thin sliced celery
- ✓ Shredded or Shaved carrot, or use vegetable peeler to make long thin slices

CONCORD SALAD DRESSING

- ✓ 1/4 cup Good Extra Virgin Olive Oil
- ✓ 1/4 cup Fresh Squeezed Lemon Juice or Red Wine Vinegar
- ✓ 1-2 tsp dijon mustard and/or a tsp of honey
- ✓ Pinch of Sea Salt & Pepper

Put all in a Jar and shake ingredients for your dressing

Bless this bowl of color and crunch
— may each bite nourish the heart, calm the gut, and awaken the soul.

This lettuce is so hydrating, fiber-rich apple, heart-healthy avocado, mineral-packed sunflower seeds, detoxifying red onion, creamy goat cheese for calcium and protein, and crunchy celery and carrot to support digestion and immunity.

CAESAR SALAD FROM THE CAPE

My friend Jen whipped this up on a visit, I was so impressed by how simple and tasty it is. This salad is now a staple meal in our home. The dressing is a bold, nourishing blend—rich in heart-healthy fats from EVOO, immune-boosting garlic, calcium-packed Parmesan, omega-3-rich anchovies, and fresh lemon to brighten digestion and detox.

DRESSING INGREDIENTS

- ✓ 1 cup of great quality extra virgin olive oil
- ✓ 1/2 c of fresh squeezed lemon juice (about 2-3 lemons)
- ✓ About 3-4 cloves of garlic, smashed to remove skins
- ✓ 1 can of anchovy filets
- ✓ 2 tsp dijon mustard
- ✓ Pinch of ground pepper
- ✓ 1/2 cup grated Parmesan

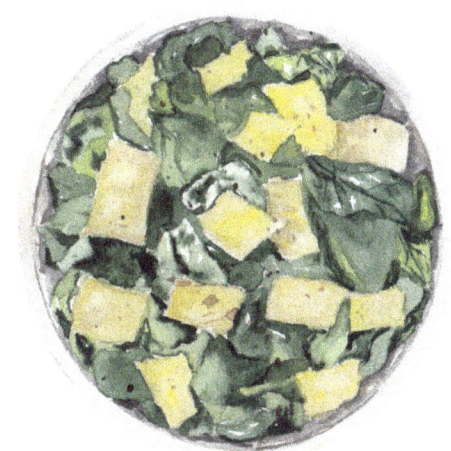

Put everything (except the cheese) in a blender or mini processor until smooth and then add cheese, whip it for another few seconds and you're done!
Serve over chopped Romaine Lettuce and Sourdough croutons - add Grilled Chicken to make it a meal.
Chop Organic Romaine Lettuce into 1" pieces, wash in a salad spinner, making sure to dry as much as possible.
Just grill or toast slices of Sourdough bread for a few seconds on each side, cut into ½-1" cubes.
Toss all, with love, to combine in a large salad bowl. Sprinkle some shaved parmesan on top.

SUMMER SALAD

If you really want easy summer nights, that's what you get when you whip up this summer salad. This is a light and zesty bowl — may its brightness lift your mood, its simplicity bring peace, and its goodness nourish you with every golden bite.

INGREDIENTS

- ✓ Fresh Squeezed Juice from 2 Lemons (about 1/4 cup)
- ✓ EVOO about 1/4 cup
- ✓ Sea Salt
- ✓ Fresh Cracked Pepper
- ✓ Fresh Grated Parmesan Cheese

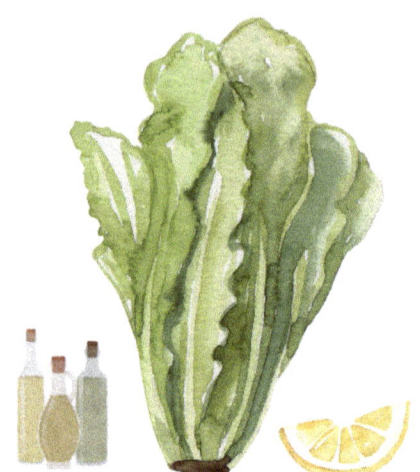

In a one to one ratio, mix fresh squeezed lemon juice and good quality EVOO with a little salt and pepper in a jelly jar. Shake it up.
Pour over chopped romaine, (mixed greens, arugula or whatever you scored from the local farmers market).
Toss to dress and add grated Parmesan to your liking.
Serve with Burgers or Grilled Chicken

YUMMY KALE SALAD !!!

Bill's Aunt Susan is a Registered Dietitian. She is always good to bring a veggie platter for family gatherings. Thanks, Aunt Sue! She recently brought over the best kale salad that I have ever had!

The secret is in the light dressing and balance of ingredients sweet and savory which delivers fiber-rich kale and carrots for digestion, antioxidant-packed berries for cell protection, red onion for detox support, and almonds for heart-healthy fats and satisfying crunch—all in one healing, colorful bowl. You are what you eat.

INGREDIENTS

- ✓ 3 cups chopped kale
- ✓ ½ cup shredded carrots
- ✓ ½ cup chopped red onion
- ✓ ½ cup fresh blueberries
- ✓ 1/3 cup dried cranberries (no sugar added)
- ✓ ¼ C sliced Almonds

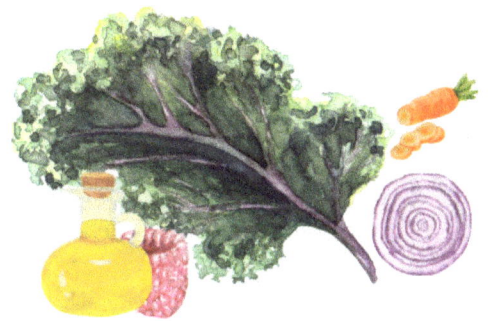
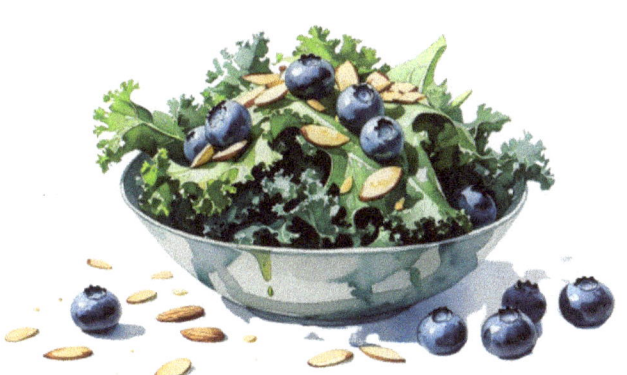

DRESSING INGREDIENTS (shake ingredients in jelly jar or whisk vigorously in a small bowl)
4T raspberry vinegar (you can always use RWV and add a teaspoon of raspberry jam)
½ cup organic grape seed oil or avocado oil ~ S&P to taste

Massage Chopped Kale with a tsp of oil and Meditate (intentional breathing) while doing so, about 2 minutes. This breaks up the kale, making it softer and easier to digest.
Toss with dressing & enjoy!

CHRISTMAS SALAD
(AND OUR TRADITIONAL CHRISTMAS MEAL)

For a no brainer, delicious Christmas meal, do this:
(and as Bill's grandfather would do, open gifts first!)

A healthy holiday meal nourishes more than the body—it balances indulgence with intention, supports energy and mood, and helps you feel joyful, not sluggish, so you can fully enjoy the celebration.

Filet Mignon on Grill, or Beef Tenderloin Roast in oven and slice
Grilled or Roasted Whole Portobello Mushrooms (marinate with EVOO & Balsamic Vinegar)
Caramelized Onions
And this Organic Mixed Greens Salad, Keep it Simple:

FOR THE SALAD
- ✓ Organic Mixed Greens
- ✓ Grapefruit segments
- ✓ crumbled gorgonzola
- ✓ sliced red onion
- ✓ S&P, try sprinkling salt and pepper on your lettuce, just like the restaurants do.

    Dressing: 1:1 ratio. RWV:EVOO, S&P

Shake in Jar and toss!

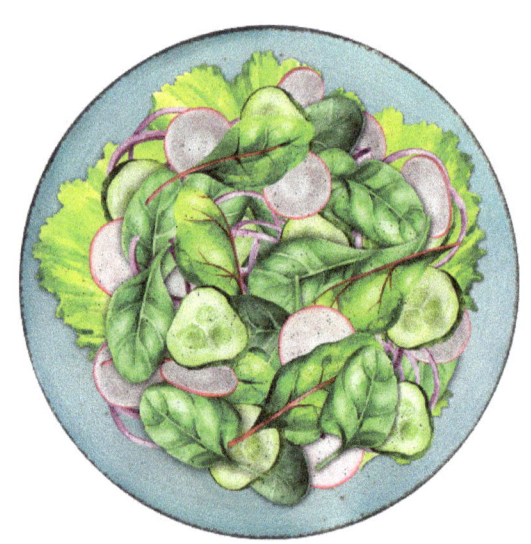

CARROT GINGER DRESSING (DIP)

This classic Japanese House Salad Dressing is mouth watering and so healthy for you, if you use the right oils! Carrots are an excellent source of vitamins, boost immunity (which we all need these days), onions promote heart health and can reduce risks of diseases! Ginger is another powerhouse - aids in digestion, promotes healthy cell growth...what are you waiting for - whip it up!

INGREDIENTS

- ✓ I C Avocado Oil
- ✓ 1/2 c rice vinegar
- ✓ 1/4 c coconut aminos
- ✓ 1T coconut sugar
- ✓ 1 1/2 T grated fresh ginger
- ✓ 2 medium chopped carrots
- ✓ 1/2 yellow chopped onion
- ✓ Sea salt & Ground pepper to taste

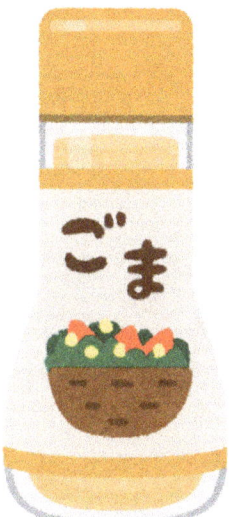

Throw it all in a powerful blender or food processor.

Note: on fresh ginger: when I find fresh (or cured) organic ginger, I stockpile it cut into 1" pieces and throw in my favorite appliance- my freezer! You can grate what you need and put it back in.

ALL IN ONE ASIAN DRESSING / DIP / MARINADE

It is a challenge to find a Food Is My Religion approved Asian Dressing, so here you go, make your own:

INGREDIENTS

- ✓ 2T Sesame Oil
- ✓ 1/2 c Organic Coconut Aminos
- ✓ 1/2 c Organic Rice Wine Vinegar
- ✓ 2T Chopped Cilantro
- ✓ 1" Fresh Ginger Grated
- ✓ 1 Garlic Clove Grated
- ✓ A few sprinkles of sesame seeds

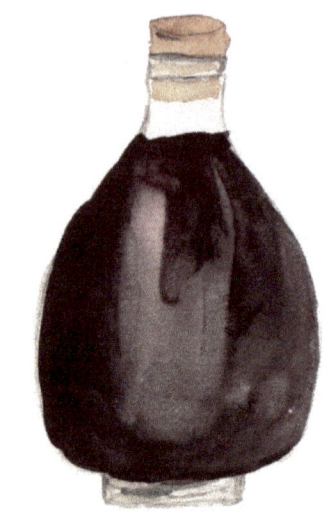

Shake all ingredients in Jar.

Add to thinly sliced cucumbers, cabbage salad, marinate chicken or sauté ground pork adding a few tablespoons to your liking. No Naughty List ingredients here!

CHIMICHURRI

This chimichurri is a vibrant, healing sauce—parsley and cilantro support detox and digestion, olive oil offers heart-healthy fats, garlic and red pepper fight inflammation, and red wine vinegar enhances nutrient absorption and gut health.

INGREDIENTS

- ✓ 1 cup (packed) fresh Italian parsley
- ✓ 1/2 cup (packed) fresh cilantro
- ✓ 1/2 cup olive oil
- ✓ 1/3 cup red wine vinegar
- ✓ 2 garlic cloves, smashed and peeled
- ✓ 1/2 teaspoon dried crushed red pepper
- ✓ 1/2 teaspoon ground cumin
- ✓ 1/2 teaspoon salt & pepper

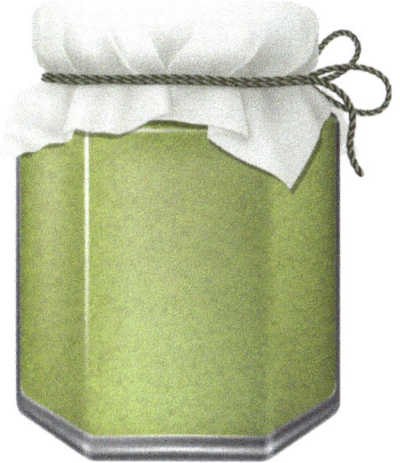

Blend all ingredients in a high powered blender, can prep ahead of time and keep room temp for 1-2 hours, or in the refrigerator up to a day before.
Serve with Marinated Skirt steak, and french fries, it's fantastic on eggs as well.

TACO SEASONING

Always thinking of tacos, and always ready to whip them up. I keep a jar of this homemade taco seasoning in my pantry. A great way to use your spices, you know what's going on your plate and in your mouth.

You can mix 1 Tbsp of this mix with 1Tbsp water or directly sprinkle it on beef or turkey chopmeat, cubed or shredded chicken to make a quick taco filler….

TACO SEASONING

   (Add all ingredients to a jar and mix well. Store in a jar and use whenever you feel like tacos)

- ✓ 4 tbsp chili powder
- ✓ 1 tsp garlic powder
- ✓ 1 tsp onion powder
- ✓ 1 tsp crushed red pepper flakes
- ✓ 1 tsp oregano
- ✓ 2 tsp paprika
- ✓ 4 tsp cumin
- ✓ 4 tsp salt
- ✓ 4 tsp black pepper

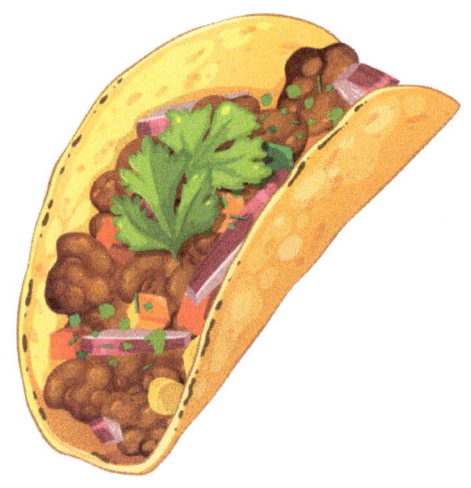

MANGO SALSA

Mango is great for your skin, reduces inflammation, great for your immune system by offering Vitamin A & Vitamin C.

I often buy the pre-cut mango and use my trusty chopper to make even cubes

FEEL FREE TO MEASURE WITH YOUR HEART HERE...

- ✓ 2 Ripe Mangos Diced
- ✓ 1 Small Red Onion diced (or shallot)
- ✓ ½-1 Jalapeno
- ✓ 1/4 C cilantro chopped
- ✓ 1-2T Avocado oil
- ✓ 1 Lime juiced
- ✓ S&P to taste

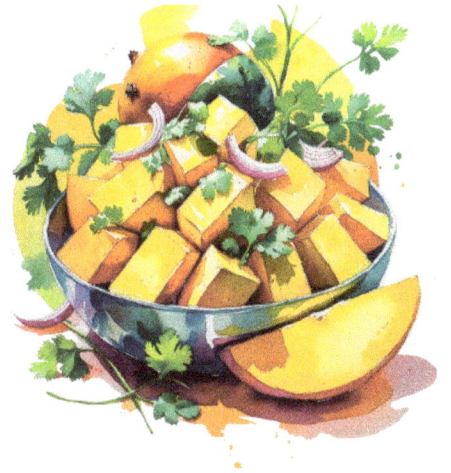

Mix all ingredients and drizzle Avocado oil.

HOMEMADE TZATZIKI & CUCUMBER TOMATO SALAD

Created to serve alongside the Mediterranean Meatballs, these dips and salad can be a great appetizer accompaniment to hummus, gluten free crackers, sliced cucumbers and carrots.

HOMEMADE TZATZIKI

- 1/2 Cup Plain Greek Yogurt
- 1 Cucumber diced
- 1 garlic clove minced (optional)
- Sprinkle of fresh squeezed lemon juice

Blend with a mini whisk and tada! No yucky ingredients here.

CUCUMBER TOMATO SALAD

- 3 C Sliced Cucumbers
- 2 C Cherry tomatoes sliced
- 1/4 red onion thin sliced
- 1/4c herbs: Fresh parsley, dill, cilantro. chives, green onion

    Whisk together:

- 4 T EVOO
- 2 T Red Wine Vinegar
- 1 t dijon mustard
- 1/4 t dried oregano
- s&p

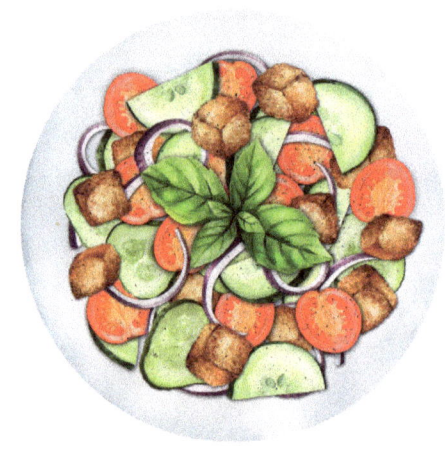

SOUPS AND STEWS

GAZPACHO

This is perfect for Labor Day weekend!! Summer Fruits of labor at work! Run to your local farmers market with this list!

INGREDIENTS
- ✓ 2 Large red tomatoes
- ✓ 2 cucumbers
- ✓ 1/4 red onion
- ✓ Handful of Cilantro (home grown, organically or local farmers market)
- ✓ 1 roasted red pepper (from a jar is fine)
- ✓ 1/3 cup Red Wine vinegar,
- ✓ 1/4 Cup good quality EVOO

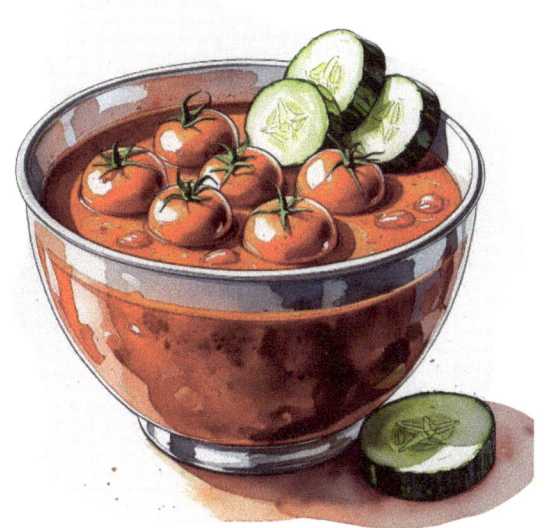

Roughly chop the 2 Large red tomatoes , 2 cucumbers, 1/4 red onion, some cilantro - throw it in your food processor with a roasted red pepper and pulse a few times to get a consistency that you like (not too much) slowly drizzle 1/3 cup Red Wine vinegar, 1/4 Cup good quality EVOO. Refrigerate for a few hours. Serve it cold on a hot day or use as a salsa - a great way to get your veggie in!

FUN Facts:
Tomatoes reduce inflammation, promotes heart health and great source of Vitamins C, A, K.
Cilantro promotes detoxification and boosts immunity.
Cucumbers are great for hydration and cooling your body, aids in weight loss, boosts skin health and supports eye health.
Onions are a superfood reducing risks of chronic illness and cancer.

CHILI - 3 WAYS

This is the best Chili Recipe - I make it EVERY Halloween, neighbors know they can come and get some after they've been trick or treating til the kids fall down. One of my favorite neighborhood traditions. I serve it with cornbread and all the toppings: Diced Red onion, shredded grass fed raw cheddar cheese and sour cream.

You can change this recipe to work for Paleo or Vegetarian (3 ways to enjoy).
You can also sub the ground beef for ground chicken or turkey for a lighter meal.

INGREDIENTS

- ✓ 1 1/4 lbs lean ground beef (For paleo: double and omit beans; for vegetarian: use 2-3 more cans of beans and omit the beef)
- ✓ 2 bell pepper diced (I love mixing colors here)
- ✓ 2 large red onions diced (reserve some for topping)
- ✓ 2 Tbs chili powder
- ✓ 2 Tbs ground cumin
- ✓ 1 tsp Worcestershire sauce (look for low sodium)
- ✓ 1 1/2 tsp salt
- ✓ 1 1/2 tsp dried oregano
- ✓ 1 1/2 tsp dried basil
- ✓ 1 tsp Tabasco

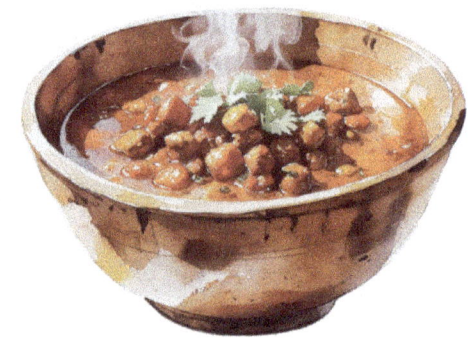

- ✓ 1/2 tsp Black pepper
- ✓ 1/4 tsp cayenne pepper
- ✓ 2 cans beans (I like to mix Black Beans and Red Kidney beans drain and rinse)
- ✓ 28oz can Good quality Crushed Tomatoes

In a large stock pot, sauté peppers and onion over medium-low heat for about 10 minutes until soft. Add ground beef and continue to brown for another 10 minutes.
Add Spices halfway through, mix well into the cooking meat or beans.
When chopmeat is no longer red, add canned tomato and beans and bring to a simmer.
Simmer for about 30 minutes to blend flavor.
Serve with toppings.

BUTTERNUT SQUASH SOUP

Perfect for a Fall Day with Toasted Pumpkin seeds as topping - nothing like a cup of Butternut Squash Soup to cozy up to Autumn. Get all the vegetable benefits and more from this warming soup: Butternut Squash, Carrots, Onion and Garlic offer immune support, reduces inflammation, adds fiber, great for eye health and heart health.

STEP 1
Roast the following on Parchment Lined Baking sheet for 40 minutes at 350°F:

- ✓ 1 Large butternut squash cubed without skin
- ✓ 4 Large carrots peeled, or washed, cut into 2" diagonal pieces
- ✓ 1 medium onion, quartered, remove outer skin
- ✓ 5 cloves garlic, crushed and peeled
- ✓ Drizzle 2 tsp avocado oil
- ✓ Drizzle 2 T Maple Syrup
- ✓ Sprinkle with Sea Salt and Pepper

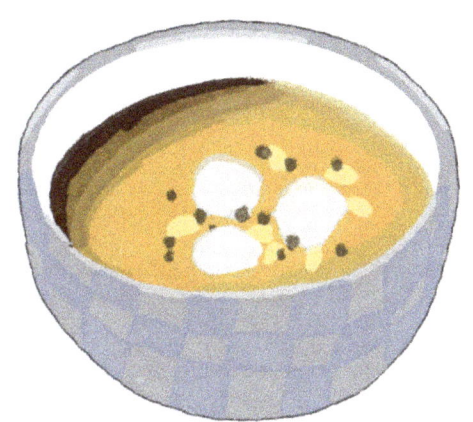

STEP 2
Then, In a large pot, add the roasted veggies with:

- ✓ 4 cups chicken or beef bone broth
- ✓ 1/4 cup half & Half or light coconut milk to make it creamy, or omit
- ✓ 1/4 tsp ground cinnamon
- ✓ 1 pinch cayenne

Let simmer for about 20 minutes. Carefully, turn off the heat to use an immersion blender to a consistency that you prefer. You can also use a high-powered blender or food processor and return to the pot.

Serve with toasted pumpkin seeds or toasted sourdough.

RAMEN (RADISH NOODLE SOUP)

After trying several recipes from blogs, Pinterest, magazines, I finally winged it - made it my own and came out the BEST! The key here is to make it your own!
Use Organic Ingredients if you can. And please add more or less of what you like!

INGREDIENTS:

- ✓ 1 Tbsp Sesame Oil
- ✓ 1/2 Onion Chopped
- ✓ 1 clove garlic
- ✓ 1 tsp ginger chopped
- ✓ 2 Quarts broth or stock of your liking (what I use: organic low sodium Chicken bone broth)
- ✓ 1 Tbsp White Miso Paste (just omit if you don't have this)
- ✓ 1/2 Cup Chopped Bok Choy
- ✓ 1/2 Cup Baby Kale rough chopped
- ✓ 1 cup Shiitake Mushrooms washed and chopped
- ✓ Any other veggie you want in there!
- ✓ 1-2 cups spiralized Daikon Radish (or separately follow directions on the package for gluten free ramen noodles and avoid all the gross seasoning packets)
- ✓ Dash of sea salt, pepper and red pepper flakes to taste
- ✓ **Toppings:** chopped cilantro and scallions and Soft Boiled egg

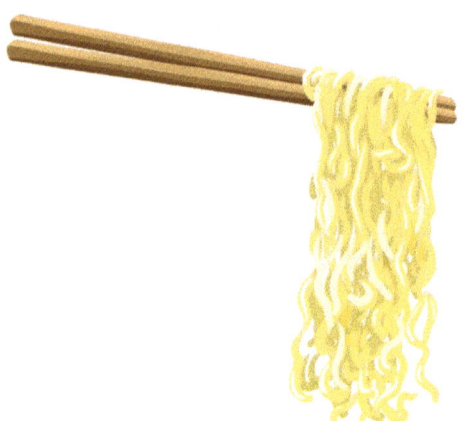

Step 1: Sauté Chopped Onion, minced garlic and ginger in Sesame Oil until softened
Step 2: Add Broth and 1 Tbsp Miso paste (I think this is the secret ingredient, but you can certainly omit - Try Miso Master Organic White Miso Gluten Free)
Bring to Boil and lower to simmer.
In a separate pot: Prepare Ramen (optional, especially if using the spiralized Radish, what I use: Organic Brown Rice Ramen found at Costco) Drain and rinse.

Step 3: Add in and simmer for 5 minutes: (These are rough estimates of add ins, seriously, add in whatever you have in fridge, whatever you like)

- ✓ 1/2 Cup Chopped Bok Choy
- ✓ 1/2 Cup Baby Kale rough chopped
- ✓ 1 cup Shiitake Mushrooms washed and chopped
- ✓ 1-2 cups spiralized Daikon Radish
- ✓ Dash of sea salt, pepper and red pepper flakes to taste
- ✓ Top with chopped cilantro and scallions and
- ✓ Soft Boiled egg (what I do: steam eggs ahead of time for 7-8 min cool in an ice bath and keep in fridge)
- ✓ Also - Add in shredded chicken, pork belly, thinly sliced steak for extra protein punch!

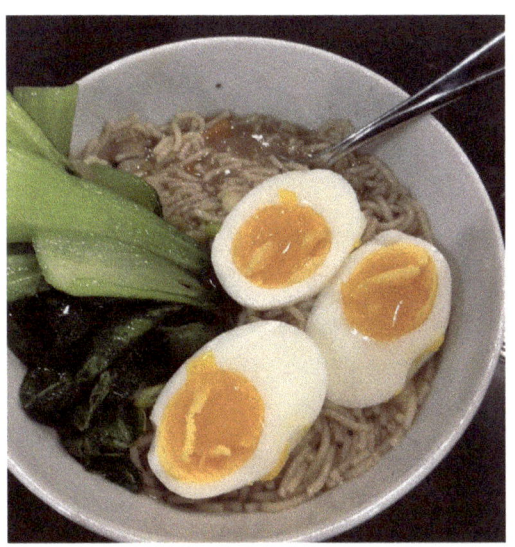
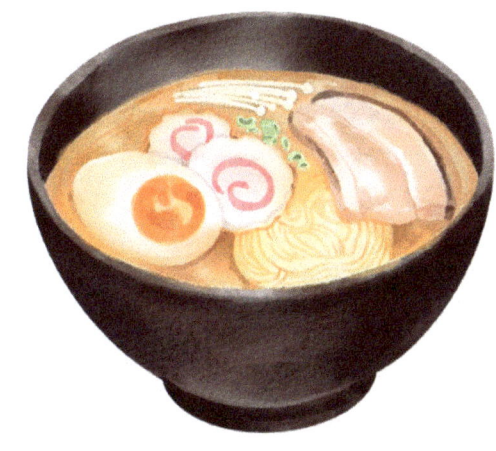

SOUPS AND STEWS

UNCLE STU'S CHICKEN NOODLE SOUP

At my nephew Gabe's Bris, I had the most amazing Matzo Ball Soup. Made by my sister in law's Uncle Stew! He says there's no "real" recipe, but here's his method:

Also known as Matzo Ball Soup…

"There is no recipe, just add ingredients & hope for the best" (I think this is a great motto and really appreciate you sharing, Uncle Stu!). It's not hard, and so worth it; also known as Jewish Penicillin. So….here goes:

PREP CHICKEN AND BROTH

Starting with the chicken, Use bone in chicken parts, thighs, legs, wings or use a whole chicken. Place chicken, carrots, celery, onion, a few garlic cloves and a bay leaf, sea salt and peppercorns in a large pot and fill with water about 2" above the chicken. Bring to a boil. Once the water is boiling, reduce heat to low. Let simmer for about an hour & then fork the chicken to determine if it is soft and will break apart.

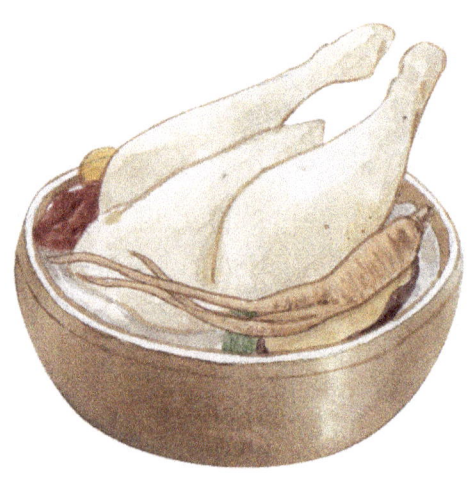

At this time, remove chicken from the pot and put in a large bowl. Pull apart the meat from the chicken, & place the bones back in the pot, continue to boil for another hour. (this becomes your broth)

MAKE THE SOUP

After an hour, Drain the pot with bones and all - a reserve liquid to add back into the pot - discard the bones and veggies, etc.
At this point, add the following ingredients to taste:
Add the fresh bite size chopped vegetables to the pot of soup.

- ✓ 1. Fresh carrots
- ✓ 2. Celery
- ✓ 3. Cooking onions

Let the soup stew in the covered pot for a couple of hours. (You can add some more store bought broth if you need more stock..
The soup should take on the color of chicken soup & smell like chicken soup.

PREPARE THE MATZO BALLS

Next, I prepare the matzo balls. For this, I use a box of Matzo meal, follow directions on the box. I prepare the matzo balls to boil in their own pot of water. As per the instructions on the box, make sure to roll 'small' balls, as they do grow in the water.

FINAL STEPS

When this is finished, place the matzo balls, shredded chicken back to the stock. Continue to sample the soup as time passes, and add seasoning that suits your taste. Depending upon how much chicken you start with, the process should take between 3-4 hours.

When cooled sufficiently, place in the refrigerator. When the soup has chilled, the fat will jell at the top. Skim off as much of the fat as you can.

"Good luck & hope you like……..save me some."

MAIN COURSES

BAKED CHICKEN CUTLETS

While we like a variety of protein sources, this chicken recipe is a staple in our house. You can slice it for sandwiches, chop it for salads and since every other day is Taco Tuesday, Rice and bean bowls Thursday, Friday and Saturdays too.

- ✓ 4lbs boneless/skinless Chicken Cutlet Breasts (Preferably from a local poultry farm source, free range and organic fed,)
- ✓ 2 eggs
- ✓ 2 Tbsp Apple Cider Vinegar
- ✓ Gluten Free Breadcrumbs (I love Aleia's)
- ✓ EVOO (That's Extra Virgin Olive Oil)

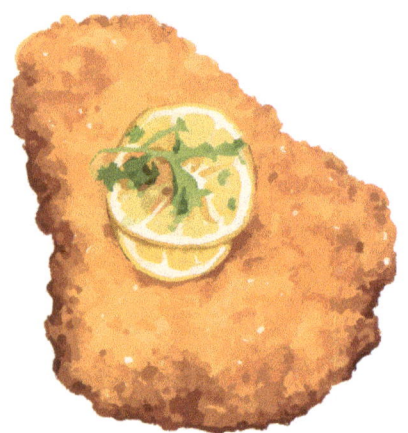

Pre-heat oven to 400°F. Crack 2 eggs in large bowl and whisk with ACV, generously season with salt and pepper.
From the chicken farm, I slice each breast into 2 thinner cutlets, or you can make 3 smaller pieces: cut the tenderloin part and then slice through the breast to get two equal size palm size pieces. Experiment here with what you love.
Spray (rub) baking sheet, lined with parchment, with a light layer of EVOO.
Lay breadcrumbs on a plate or pie dish.
One by one, take the chicken out of the egg mixture, run your hands over to get it as dry as you can and dip into breadcrumbs, press down on each side and lay on the oiled pan.
Drizzle EVOO over top and bake on the lowest rack in your oven for about 12-15 minutes each side. (Typically I do 15 minutes on the first side and 10 on the other.) The bottom of my oven gets hotter, so if you have more than one tray, you can rotate them around, after the bottoms are golden brown, flip and bake for another 12 minutes. It's not an exact science, depending on your oven. When my oven heats up it seems to go quicker. Take off pan and let air dry on cookie rack, they will stay crisper for left overs.

(Because I don't like food waste, I often use the leftover egg batter and breadcrumbs to make a modified version of the mediterranean meatballs on the following pages, another way to meal prep and keep healthy protein on hand.)

OKAL CHICKEN MARINADE

Scottie Okal is a friend, fisherman, lover of life, and teaches us to let our squid flow. Here's his Chicken Marinade recipe, which we use ALL THE TIME:

"Enough for about 8lbs. of Chicken (can be on the bone or not, we mostly do boneless breasts)....... You can marinate for two hours, marinate it for up to 24 hours (meal prep) for best taste and tenderness.

- ✓ 1 cup EVOO
- ✓ 3/4 cups soy sauce or Organic Coconut Aminos
- ✓ 1/4 cup Worcestershire sauce
- ✓ 2 tbsp dry mustard
- ✓ 1/3 cup red wine vinegar or rice vinegar
- ✓ 1 1/2 tsp chopped parsley (and/or cilantro)
- ✓ 2 crushed garlic cloves
- ✓ 1/3 cup lemon juice or red wine vinegar

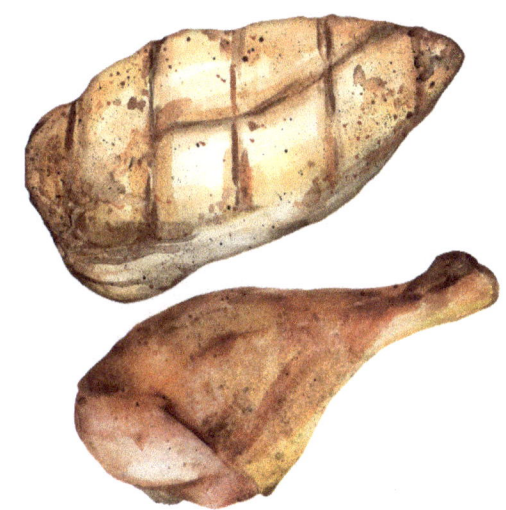

Whisk all ingredients, add chicken and let Marinate.
From the chicken farm, I slice each boneless breast into 2 thinner cutlets, or you can make 3 smaller pieces: cut the tenderloin part and then slice through the breast to get two equal size palm size pieces.
Pre Heat an outdoor grill to medium high, grill chicken 5-6 minutes each side, until an internal thermometer reaches 165°F.

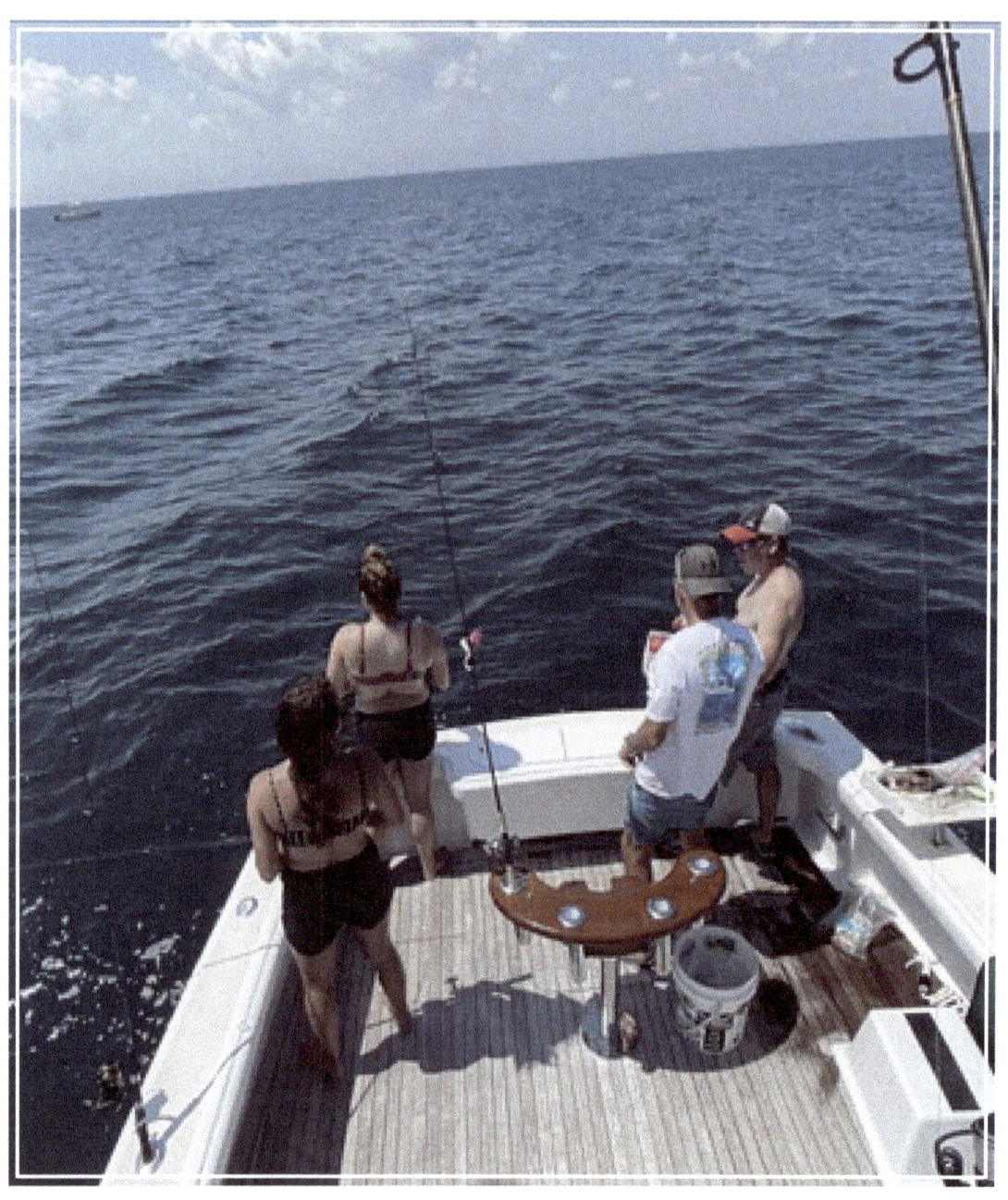

Fishing for fluke, the Okal motto reminds us to "Let your squid flow"

ROASTED LEMON CHICKEN THIGHS AND CAULIFLOWER

Aka COMING HOME MEAL

I make this meal when we've been away, when we want some healthy comfort food, and when the kids come home from college craving a home cooked meal.

- ✓ 8 Chicken thighs on the bone or combo of 4 chicken thighs and 2 breasts on bone.
- ✓ 1 Head Cauliflower, cut into 8 wedgies. (add in Carrots and/or potatoes if you want)

Whisk Marinade:

- ✓ 1/2 C EVOO
- ✓ 1-2 Tbsp Dried Thyme
- ✓ Zest of 1 Lemon, slice the lemon after zested
- ✓ S&P

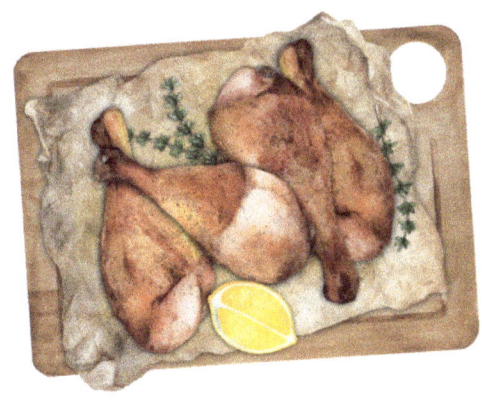
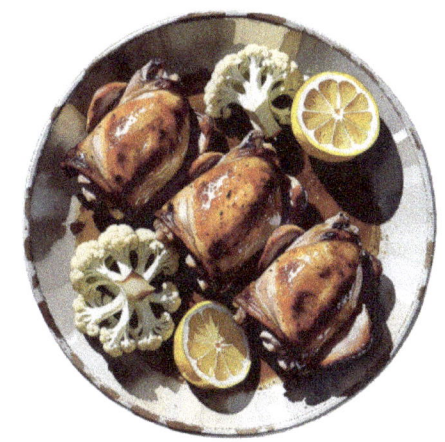

Preheat oven to 400°F.
Brush the marinade on all sides of the chicken and cauliflower.
Slice the zested lemon and lay on top of the chicken thighs, placed skin side down on a parchment lined baking sheet.
Roast for 45 minutes.
Turn skin side up and broil until crispy, 5 minutes or so.
Serve alongside the yellow rice and plantains.
Dollop of organic sour cream, chopped cilantro (get that variety of herbs in), and your favorite hot sauce.

MEDITERRANEAN MEATBALLS

A friend of mine made these small appetizer sizes and they were soooo good, full of protein and vegetables! Serve with homemade Tzatziki and Cucumber Tomato Salad.

- ✓ 1 1/4 pounds ground turkey
- ✓ 1 cup spinach, kale or Swiss chard - Finely chopped
- ✓ 1/4 cup breadcrumbs (I like them GF)
- ✓ 2 teaspoons ground cumin
- ✓ 2 cloves garlic, minced
- ✓ 1 medium carrot, grated
- ✓ 1 egg
- ✓ Sea salt and pepper

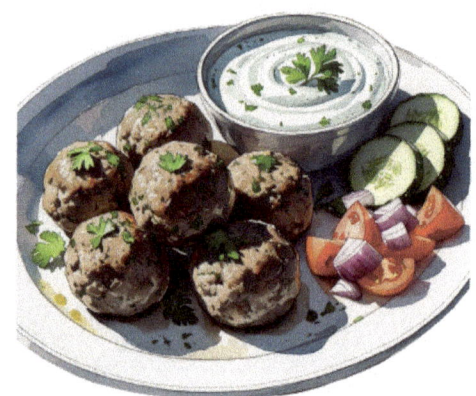

Preheat the oven 400°F. Line a baking sheet with parchment paper and drizzle Avocado Oil and spread it around with your hands. Shape Meatballs (1-2T per ball).
Space evenly on the baking sheet. Bake until cooked through, turning 1x half way through. About 12 to 14 minutes.

Meanwhile, make your dips (hummus and tzatziki) and cucumber salad to serve with.
Fill some pitas or have them in a bowl with rice.

SKIRT STEAK MARINADE

This recipe is great for up to 3 lbs of Skirt Steak (6 people), you can always double or do math X1.5. It gets gobbled up by even the pickiest of eaters, so when in doubt, make more. It's great cold, in salads or the next morning with eggs.

INGREDIENTS
- ✓ 1/2 cup coconut aminos
- ✓ 2 tablespoons honey
- ✓ 2 tablespoons rice vinegar
- ✓ 2 tablespoons sesame oil
- ✓ 2 tablespoons sesame seeds
- ✓ 2 cloves minced garlic
- ✓ 1 (1 inch) piece fresh ginger, grated
- ✓ 1/4 cup cold water
- ✓ 1 tablespoon tapioca flour

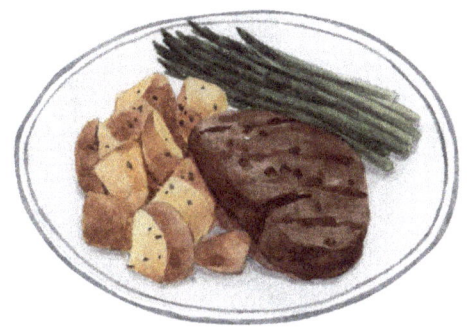

Whisk together and marinate for one hour or more, or overnight.
Grill for about 4 minutes each side.

SPRING VEGETABLE FRITTATA

A fan favorite - skip the crust, make it easy on yourself. You can whip this up when you have unexpected guests... or 25 of your husband's cousins sleep over (Hello McCuzins!)...

Eggs contain heart healthy Omega-3 fatty acids, improves brain function, and serves as a great source of selenium and protein. Also amazing as breakfast for dinner.

INGREDIENTS

- ✓ 1 Tbsp EVOO
- ✓ 1 Tbsp Grass Fed Butter
- ✓ 6-8 Fresh Asparagus Stalks trimmed and cut on diagonal into ½-1" pieces
- ✓ 2 Cups Chopped Fresh Broccoli (do this ahead of time, see notes why!)
- ✓ ½ Onion sliced thin
- ✓ 8 Eggs, whisked until fluffy
- ✓ Shredded Parmesan Cheese
- ✓ S&P to taste

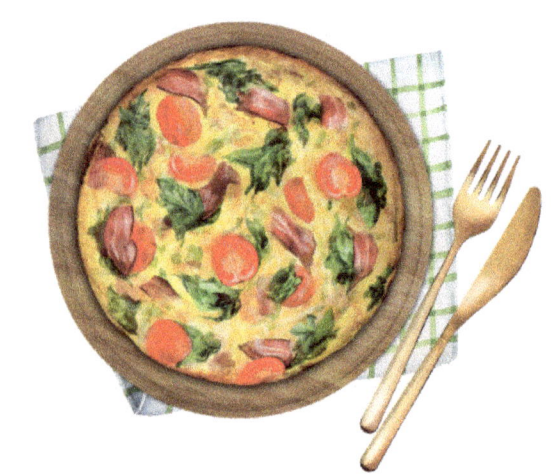

Preheat the oven to 400°F.
Sauté Vegetables: Heat 1 tablespoon of the oil in an ovenproof pan over medium-high (No plastic handles). Add the asparagus and onion, cook, stirring occasionally, until softened, about 3 minutes, add broccoli and continue to sauté about 5 minutes. While Veggies are cooking,
Whisk eggs until light and fluffy with 1 tsp sea salt, and ½ teaspoon of the pepper. Add 1 Tbsp Grass Fed Butter to the pan and mix into veggies coating the pan. Pour eggs over the vegetables in the skillet and cook, stirring gently, until the eggs just begin to set, about 1-2 minutes. Sprinkle some parmesan over the top and transfer the pan to the oven.
Bake until the center is set, 10 to 12 minutes.
Serve alongside Land of Nutrition's Baby Greens Salad everyday salad, garnish with fresh herbs: Tarragon, Chives (including a favorite - Chive flowers).

Bonus: When you chop broccoli ahead of time (40-45 minutes), and let it rest before cooking, you're performing a ritual that unlocks powerful nutrients like sulforaphane, a compound known for its detoxifying and disease-fighting powers, making it even better for your body. Remember to do this for all of your broccoli recipes.

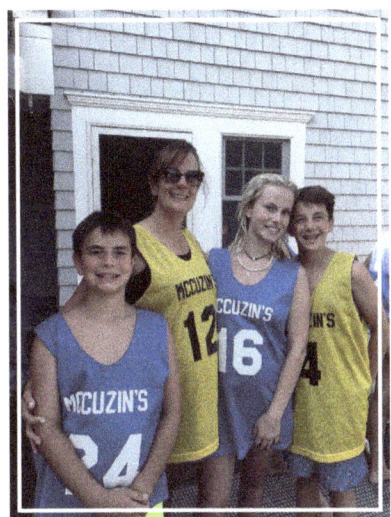
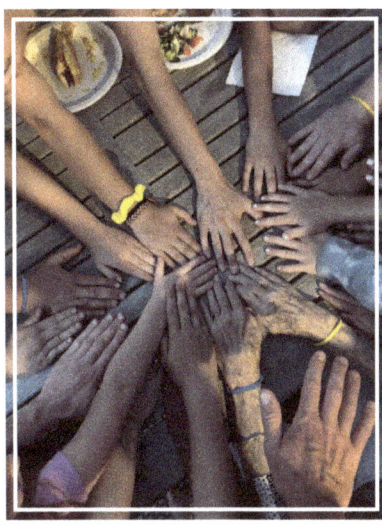
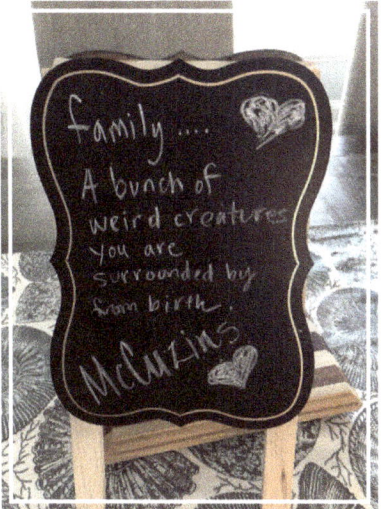

BABY LAMB CHOP DRY-ISH MARINADE - EASTER APP OR CHARMED LIFE TAILGATING

Really, my husband makes these little finger food nuggets of joy at football tailgates, easy to grill, easy to cut and easy to eat with your fingers. Get your protein variety - by adding these baby lamb chops, you get a great source of iron, zinc and vitamin B12

INGREDIENTS

- ✓ 2T Fresh Chopped Rosemary (or dried rosemary)
- ✓ 2 Large Garlic Cloves, minced
- ✓ 1 t sea salt
- ✓ 1t freshly ground pepper
- ✓ Finely grated zest of 1 lemon or lime
- ✓ 1T EVOO

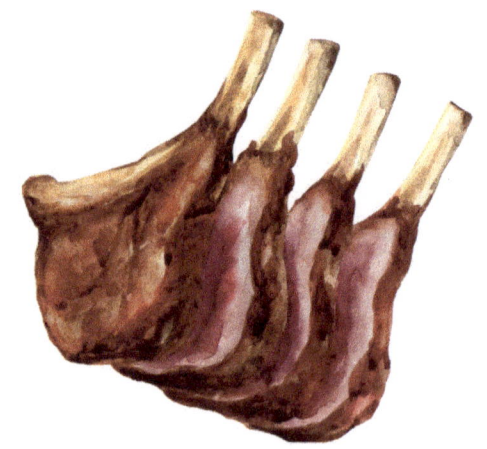

Lay foil out double layer and spread ingredients into a rack of baby lamb chops, drizzle with EVOO.

Fire up an outdoor grill on high and place the foil packet on grill for 10-15 minutes per side Carefully open the packet and slice chops into individual pieces. Place back on the grill for a few minutes to crisp edges.

Serve warm! Enjoy!

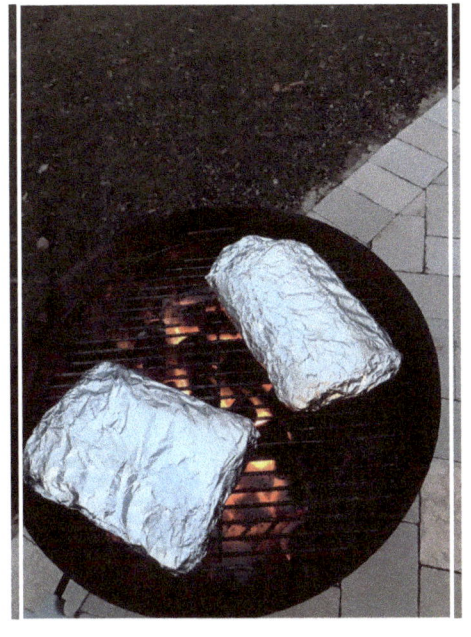
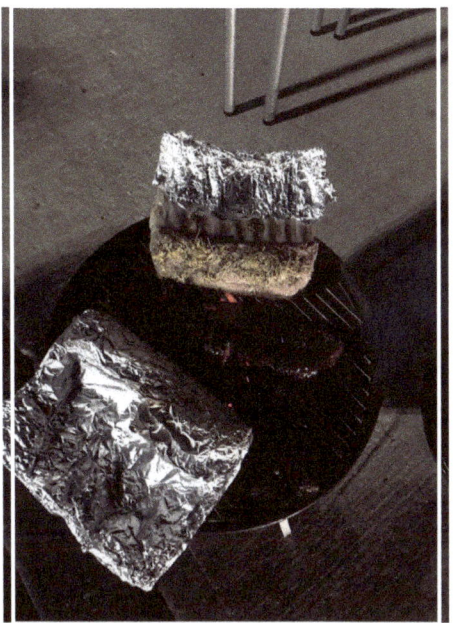
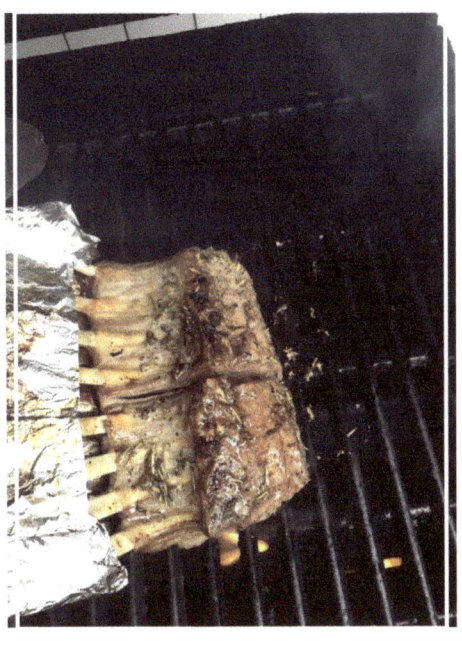
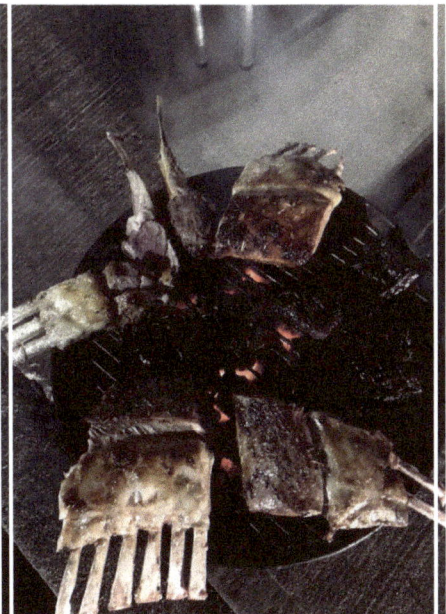

MAIN COURSES PAGE 141

GRASS FED BEEF BURGERS

The BEST Burger recipe. Period. Grass Fed Beef is best, for reasons explained in part 1 of this book, but mostly the taste is unrivaled.

INGREDIENTS
- ✓ 1 lb Quality Organic Grass Fed Beef
- ✓ 1 Tbsp Dijon Mustard
- ✓ 1 Tbsp Low Sodium Worcestershire sauce or coconut aminos
- ✓ S&P to taste

Mix well by hand, divide into 4 burgers

Grill on high heat until the middle of the burger temperature reaches 140-145 about 6 minutes per side.
My favorite way to eat burgers is on an English Muffin, but serve on roll of choice or have a burger on a salad!

Favorite topping include: Caramelized Onion, Lettuce, Avocado, and Spicy Pickle Chips, Ketchup, Mayo and Mustard

HOT DOGS

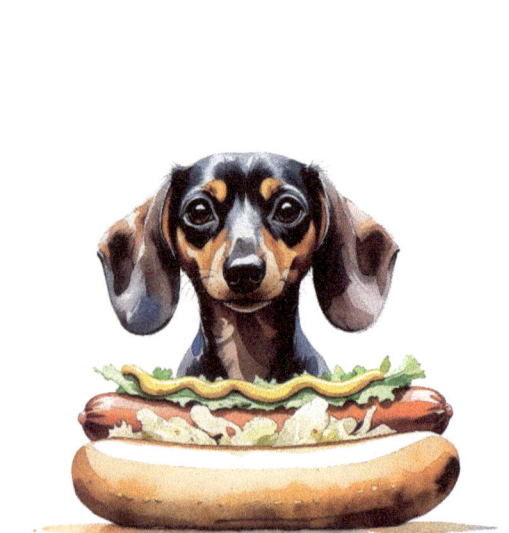

It is so easy to find "Organic Grass Fed Beef Hot Dogs" and you can tell the difference in how your body will react to this healthy alternative. Practice reading the ingredients.
Serve with Gut Healthy Sauerkraut (homemade for bonus points, see recipe)!

STRIPETOBER

The next few fish dishes are inspired by my husband, Bill. He catches Striped Bass right from the beach, the joy in his face when he reels it in is the BEST, second best is the fresh ceviche we make with it:

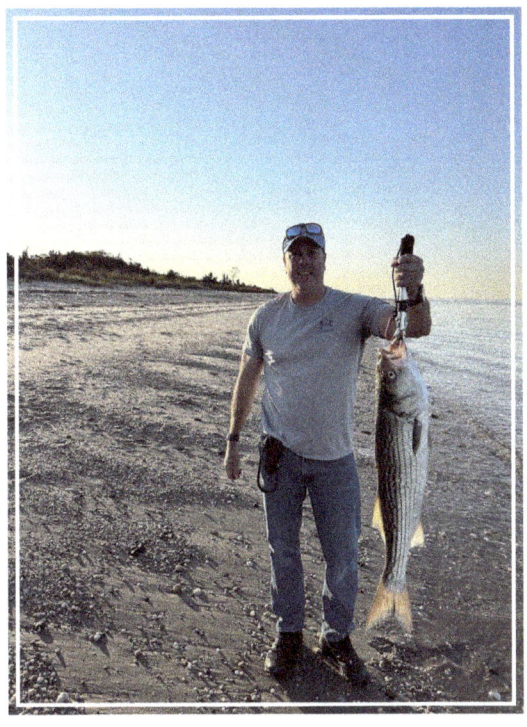
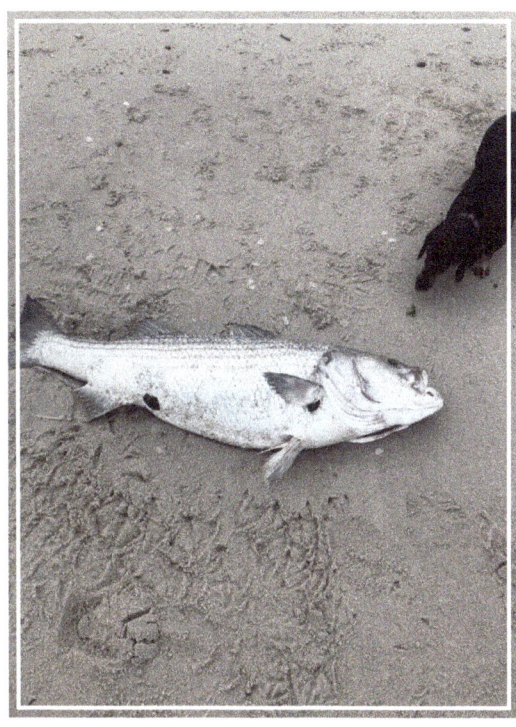

FRESH STRIPED BASS CEVICHE

Marinate bite size pieces of sushi grade fish with lime.
Add Mango, cucumber, avocado, red onion, jalapeño and cilantro.
(You can make the Mango Salsa Recipe from this book and marinate the striped bass in the juices)

Leave in the fridge for an hour or 2, season with salt and pepper and serve with chips - we love Siete Dip Chips.

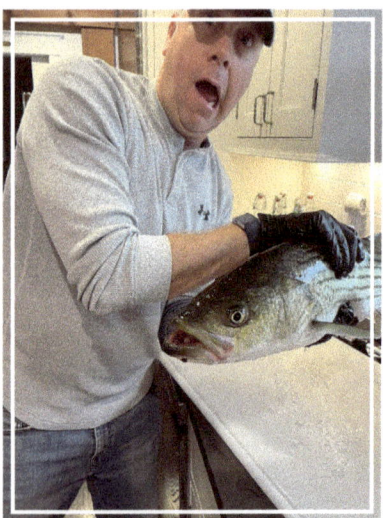
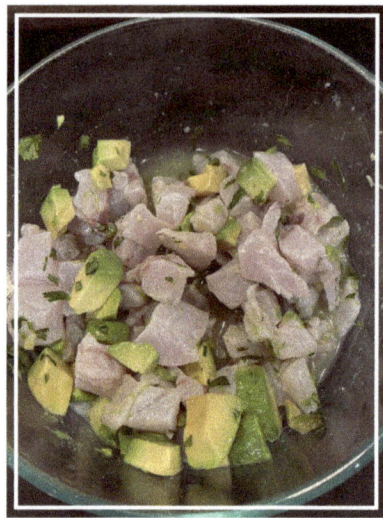
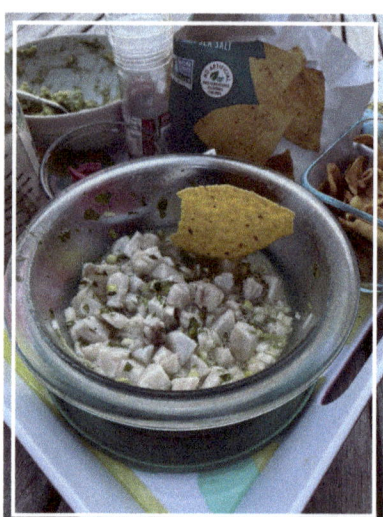

TNT FISH TACO

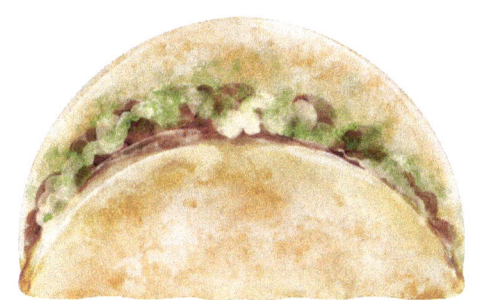

This recipe dates back to one of my first experiences in the kitchen. Great for fish tacos or to serve alongside a summer salad. The leftovers are amazing on a salad the next day.

- ✓ 1lb Striped Bass, Tilapia, flounder, or any meaty white fish

Whisk together:

- ✓ 2T AP Flour, Almond flour (or omit)
- ✓ 2T Cornmeal
- ✓ 1T Chili Powder
- ✓ 2t cumin
- ✓ 2t crushed red pepper
- ✓ 2t paprika
- ✓ 1t sea salt
- ✓ 1/2t black pepper

Dry Fish with paper towels. In a shallow dish dip fish to coat in dry mixture.
Fry in Avocado Oil for 4-6 minutes each side.
Serve over cabbage slaw or make tacos!
Don't forget the pickled onions and mango salsa.

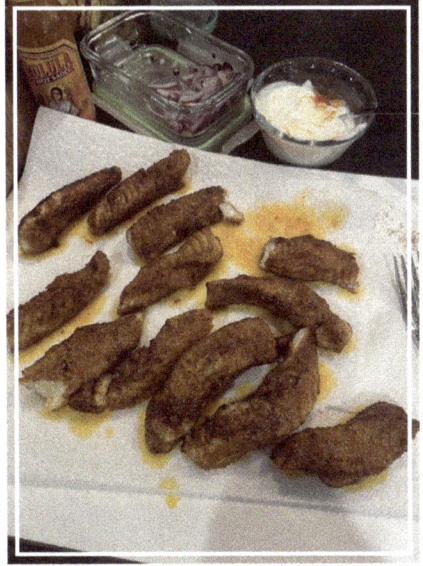
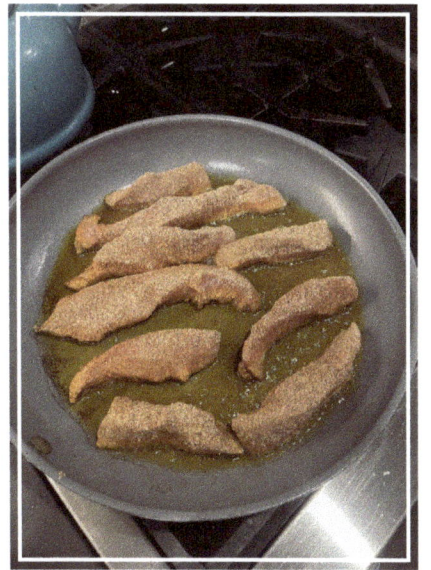

CAPE COD COD

Another classic "recipe" I learned from our friends on Cape Cod. In High School Marine Biology Class, every Friday was assigned to a student to bring in a "fish dish." While I probably didn't appreciate it then (I made a tuna salad from a can), the health benefits from fish are amazing. Light & fresh, a great source of protein, I wish I could go back in time and show off these fresh catches (recipes).

INGREDIENTS

- ✓ 1 Large Cod Fillet (We also do this with Striped Bass)
- ✓ 2T Grass fed unsalted butter
- ✓ Panko Breadcrumbs
- ✓ Garlic Powder and Montreal Seasoning
- ✓ A smidge of white wine (Optional)
- ✓ You need 1 Large Cod Fillet, melt butter and brush both sides of the fish.

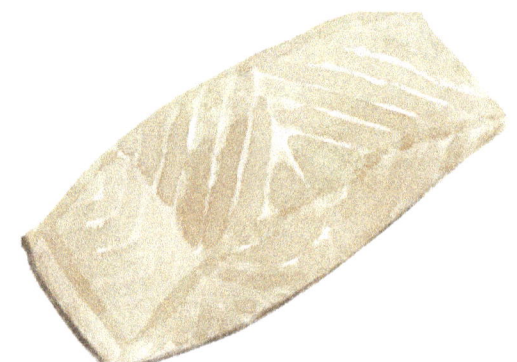

Lay in a baking dish, pour some white wine over the top.
Bake at 400ºF for about 10 minutes.
Take out and spread Panko Breadcrumbs mixed with a little garlic powder and Montreal seasoning, bake for another 10 minutes. As soon as it starts to flake, it's done baking,
Broil the top for a few minutes to brown the top.

Quick Montreal Seasoning (mix in jar and keep on hand)
2T Kosher Salt
2T Black Pepper
2T Paprica
1T Garlic Powder
1 T Onion Powder
2t coriander powder
2t dried mustard powder
1T red pepper flakes

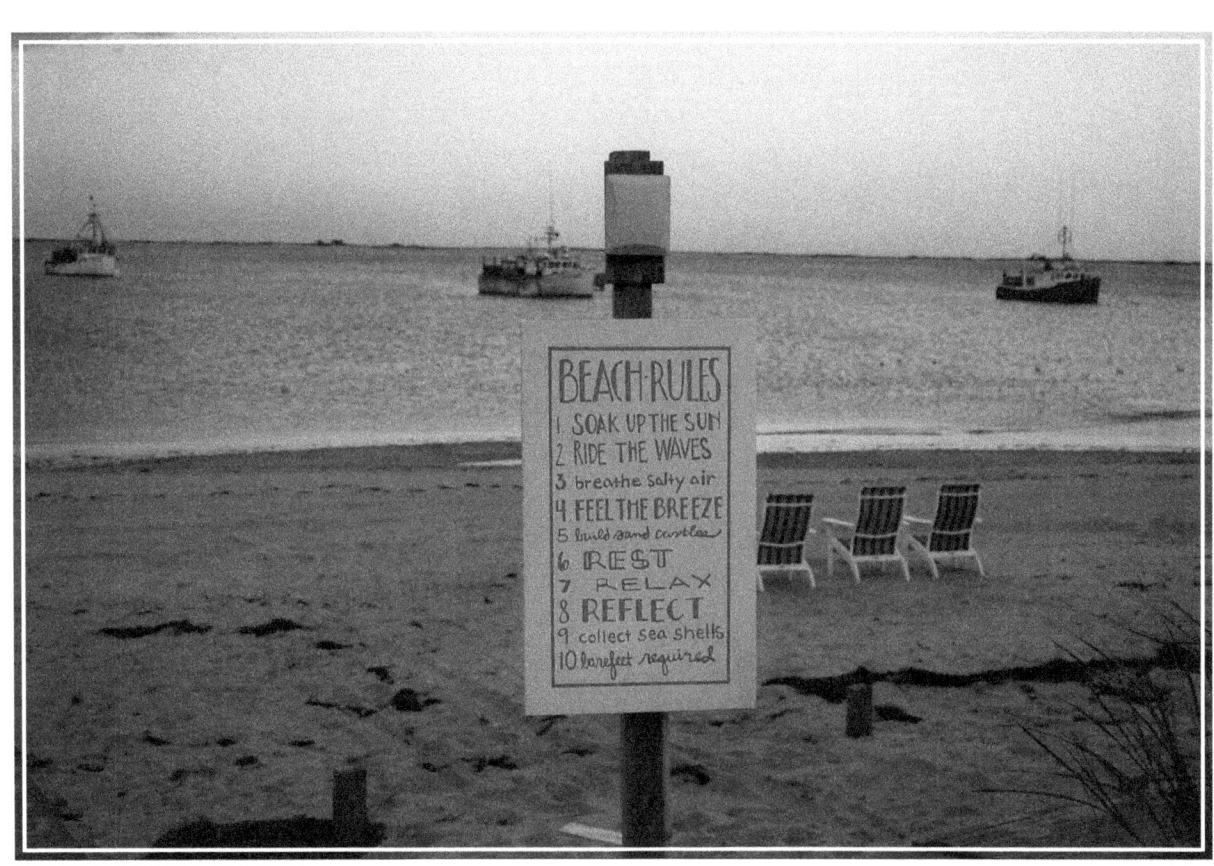

HOLIDAY BRISKET

My Grandmother made this classic with onion soup mix. In her defense, back then it probably didn't include the "Naughty List" ingredients, so I'm cleaning it up. You can absolutely do this same day as well.

The day before your holiday: Take a "1st cut" thin Brisket, season with sea salt, pepper and paprika, onion powder, garlic powder and put into a baking pan with a thinly sliced yellow onion. Add 1 cup water or broth to the pan. (Option to sear the seasoned brisket in a cast iron skillet to get a nice brown char on each side to add flavor before adding onion and water).
Bake 350°F for 2-2 1/2 hours, adding more water if necessary.
Remove, cool, put in a glass pyrex to store overnight.
Drain and reserve liquid into a jar -refrigerate overnight.

The next day: Slice brisket on an angle against the grain.
Cut 4-6 potatoes, into 1-2" chunk, place around the brisket in a baking pan.
Add the reserved liquid and 1 can crushed tomato or Land of Nutrition (no Naughty Ingredients or non-dairy) Tomato Soup.
Bake for 1 hour or until potatoes are soft.

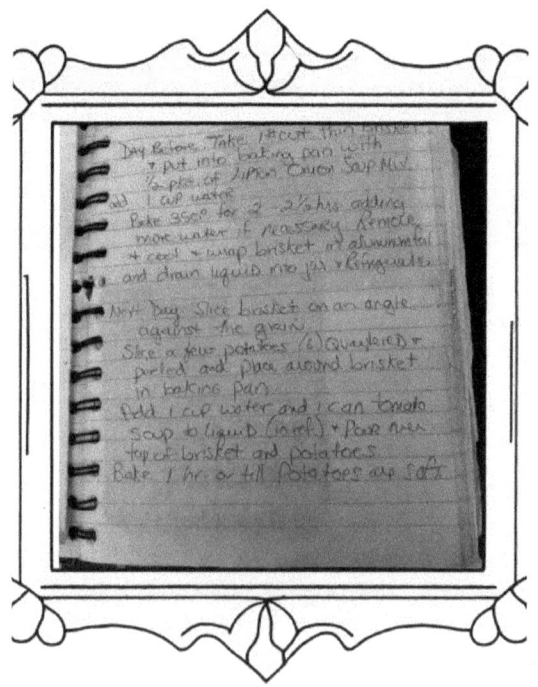

On the Side - Side Dishes

CARAMELIZED ONION

This makes a sweet addition to salads, omelets, any asian dish, onion is a superfood that boosts your immune system, reduces risk of disease and great for heart health. This take is simple and tasty. You can also add mushrooms at the end for about 5-10 minutes to make it even more healthy and hearty.

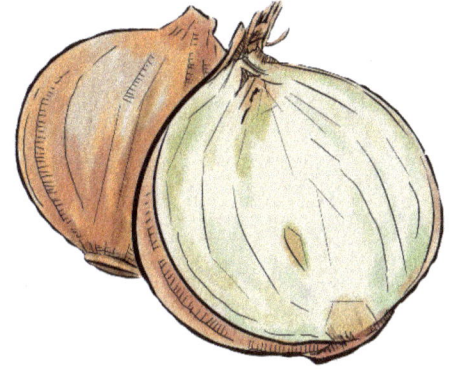

Thinly Slice Organic Yellow onions (you can also use red or white if that is what you have).

To a skillet pan, drizzle 1T of EVOO or AVO oil (I often use Ghee), add onion and sauté, stirring often for about 10 minutes. Once the onions become soft, add 1-2 Tbsp of Balsamic Vinegar for bright color and flavor. Sauté another 10 minutes and that's it!

These are also great to make a tasty soup, just add to organic beef or chicken bone broth and bring to a simmer.

QUICK PICKLED ONIONS

Pickled Onions are a great addition to salads, avocado toast or quinoa bowls.

BRING TO SIMMER:
- ✓ 1/2C Water
- ✓ 1/4 distilled white vinegar
- ✓ 1/4c apple cider vinegar
- ✓ 1 1/2T Maple Syrup
- ✓ 1 1/2t Sea Salt
- ✓ 1/4t Red Pepper Flakes

Meanwhile, Thinly slice 1 1/2 Red onion and fill a 2 cup mason jar.
Pour liquid over onion.
Bring to room temperature, cover and refrigerate.
Top tacos, salads, or quinoa bowls with egg, salsa and avocado.

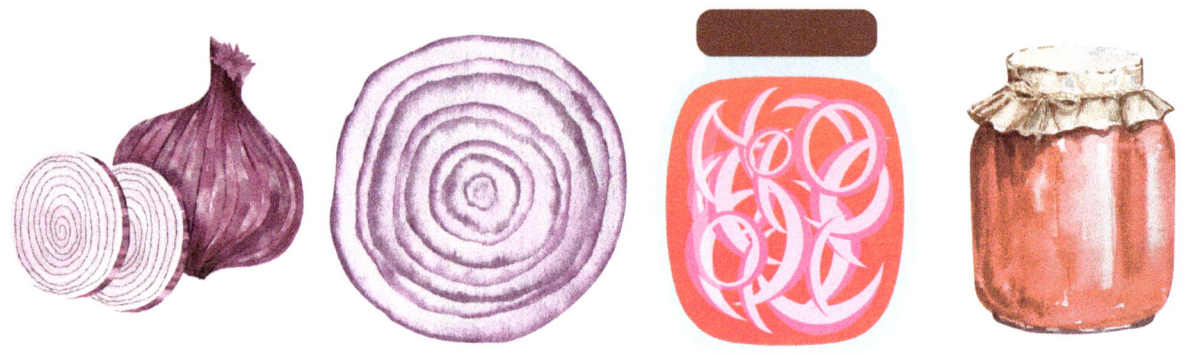

SAUTEED GREEN BEANS

When farmers markets are loaded with green beans and fresh herbs, it's prime time - so this recipe provides the perfect summer night accompaniment to skirt steak and chimichurri, using the best of what nature has intended! Get your greens in.

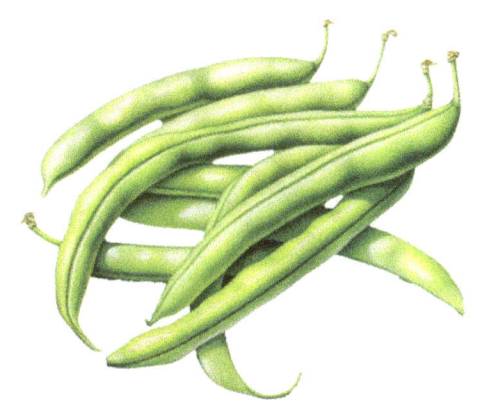

1 Bunch of Organic Green Beans (washed and trimmed)
2-4 cloves of garlic - smashed (or more, I love garlic)

Heat EVOO or Avocado Oil on low heat and add smashed garlic for a few minutes until fragrant, don't burn. Then add Green beans and sauté until desired crispness, typically 6-7 minutes.

Another bonus: Just like chopping broccoli releases more goodness, when you smash garlic ahead of time (just 10 minutes!), it activates allicin, garlic's most powerful healing compound, known for its anti-inflammatory, heart-loving, and immune-boosting benefits. So when you smash garlic with the side of a knife, it not only makes it easy to get the thin dried skin off, it adds nutrition, just do it first before you prep the greens!

HOMEMADE SAUERKRAUT

Sauerkraut is so good for you. The real kind. The fermented cabbage kind and it's so easy to make in your own kitchen!

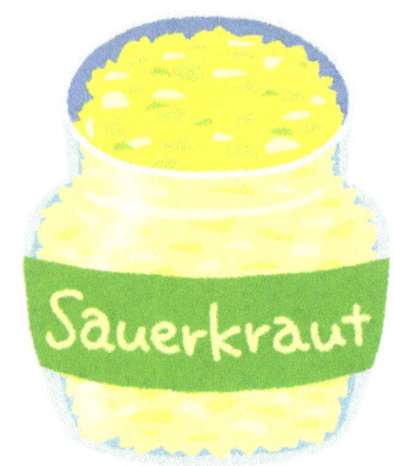

Loaded with good for your gut probiotics, sauerkraut makes a great snack, addition to salad, tacos, side gig; it can boost your immune system, improve your digestion, reduce your risk of certain diseases, it's all good if made fresh sans icky ingredients. Why not try this at home.

Sauerkraut (Fermented Cabbage) comes from the process of lacto-fermentation, transforming salt and cabbage into sauerkraut increases food enzymes and dietary fiber, vitamins B, C & K, and minerals potassium, calcium and phosphorus. This provides our bodies with beneficial probiotics, beneficial bacteria – friendly microorganisms which help to colonize the gut, train the immune system and manufacture vitamins in the digestive tract. All thanks to this natural fermentation process, this is great for our GUT health! It is so easy and fun to make!

ALL YOU NEED:

- ✓ 1 Medium Head of Organic Green Cabbage (or Red Cabbage or Mix)
- ✓ 1 Tbsp Sea Salt or Kosher Salt
- ✓ 1 32oz Canning Jar

Directions: Discard outer leaves of the cabbage (remove the next layer and keep this whole). Cut the cabbage into quarters. Thinly slice each wedge, place in a large glass mixing bowl (avoid plastic or metal), sprinkle kosher salt over the sliced cabbage.
This is a classic mediate as you chop the moment.
Massage the sliced cabbage and salt with your hands for 5–10 minutes until it becomes limp and moist. (Another opportunity for meditation).
Tightly pack the cabbage into the canning jar by tamping down with your fist or back of wooden spoon. Add any extra cabbage liquid from the bowl into the jar.
Cover completely with a large outer leaf that you saved. Make sure all cabbage is completely submerged. You can also fill a baggie with water and place on top to weigh it down or use a glass pickling weight.
Cover the jar with lid and place on the counter.

Each Day, "Burp" the lid by slightly opening it. It may let out a little gas (Burp).

Let the cabbage ferment for 3–7 days at room temperature.

Check it daily after the 4th day for desired taste. Any layer of bubbles or foam can be skimmed off during fermentation or after it's done. If you see mold, remove it immediately.

Look for color changes in the cabbage, which will go from green to yellow or deep purple to a pink. Store in the refrigerator and enjoy!

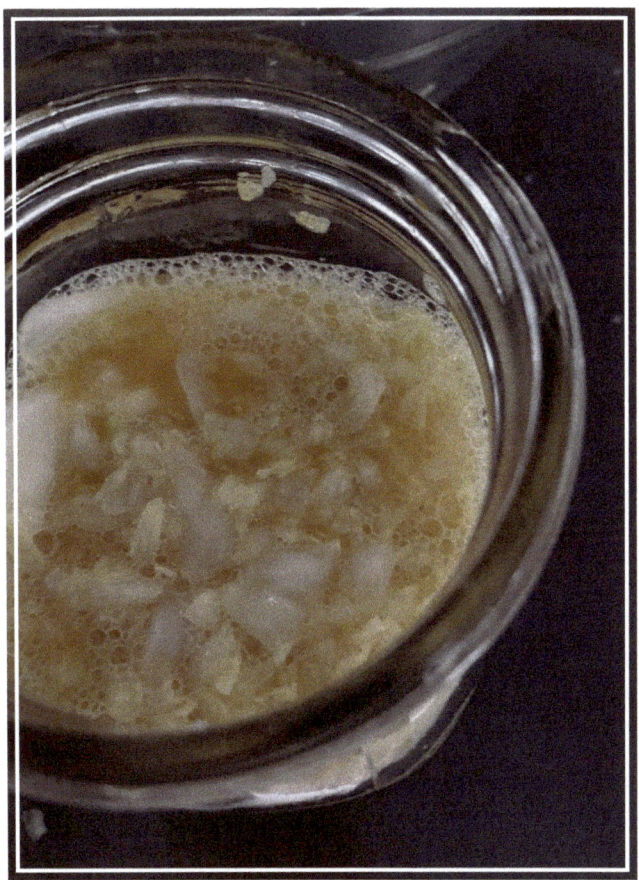

Bonus variations include: Garlic & Ginger: Add 2–3 cloves minced garlic and a thumb-sized piece of fresh ginger, grated or sliced thin, for a spicy, warming kick.

Onion & Carrot: Include ½ thinly sliced onion and 1 grated carrot for extra texture and a touch of sweetness.

Turmeric: Add about 1 to 2 teaspoons of ground turmeric (or 1 tablespoon fresh grated turmeric root) to the cabbage when you start massaging it with salt.

FRENCH FRIES AKA ROASTED POTATOES

Healthy homemade roasted potatoes, frites or french fries:

Cut potatoes to your liking and soak them in water, this will take some starch out (you will see at bottom of water) and also help the potato to crisp up.

You can do this ahead of baking - up to 2-3 hours before roasting, which is helpful when having guests. Aim for draining and drying approximately 1 hour before meal time.

Line a baking sheet with parchment paper and lightly coat with EVOO or Avo Oil. Add Potatoes in a single Layer.

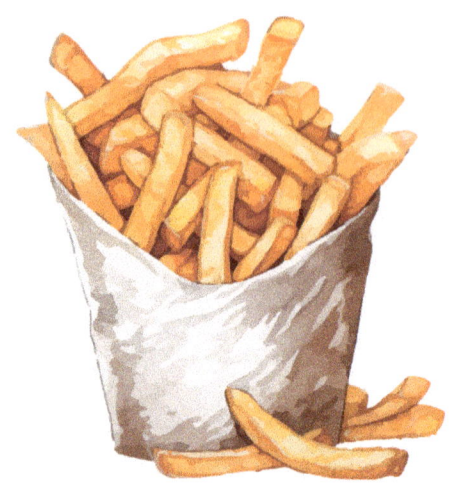

Sprinkle generously with sea salt, pepper and my secret ingredient: paprika!

Bake at 400 for about an hour, turning and flipping every 20-25 minutes until desired crispness is achieved!

Enjoy with our favorite French Fry dip: mayo and ketchup (remember read your labels)!

When potatoes cool down, the glycemic index goes down. So make more and enjoy tomorrow.

YELLOW RICE

In the 80's and 90's we ate rice out of a box, with packets of who knows what?
This method is healthier and just as easy!

INGREDIENTS

- ✓ 1 t Turmeric
- ✓ 1/2t Cumin
- ✓ 1/2t sea salt
- ✓ Pinch Cinnamon
- ✓ 1T Butter or Ghee
- ✓ 1.5 Cups Brown Rice (or any rice you have)

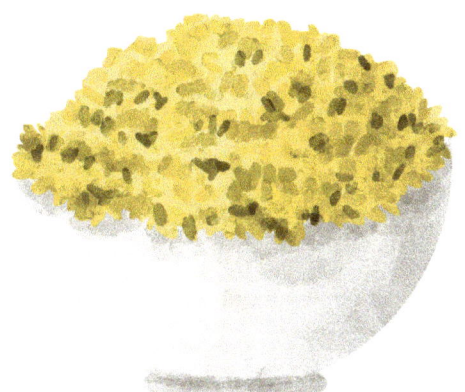

In a Medium Sized pot, heat turmeric, cumin and
cinnamon for 30 seconds, then melt 1Tbsp Grass Fed Butter or Ghee
Add 3C water, ½ tsp sea salt and Rice

Bring to boil for about 20 minutes until water is absorbed and rice is soft or to your liking.

We like to serve alongside Roasted Chicken and Cauliflower (with chopped cilantro, Organic Raw Cheddar Cheese and a dollop of organic sour cream.

BEST POTATO LATKES

We serve these at Hanukkah, especially as appetizers at our annual Latke & Vodka neighbor party. Baked, not fried and so yummy - they can be made a day in advance and reheat well.

- ✓ 2 lb Russet potatoes, cut lengthwise into quarters (Leave skins on, because who needs all that extra work?)
- ✓ 1 large yellow onion, peeled and cut into quarters
- ✓ 3 large eggs
- ✓ 1/2 cup potato starch, cassava flour or tapioca flour
- ✓ 1 tsp sea salt
- ✓ 1/4 tsp fresh ground black pepper
- ✓ 1/4 cup slightly melted ghee
- ✓ Preheat the oven to 425°F. Prepare two large baking sheets lined with parchment paper, lightly coat with AVO oil .

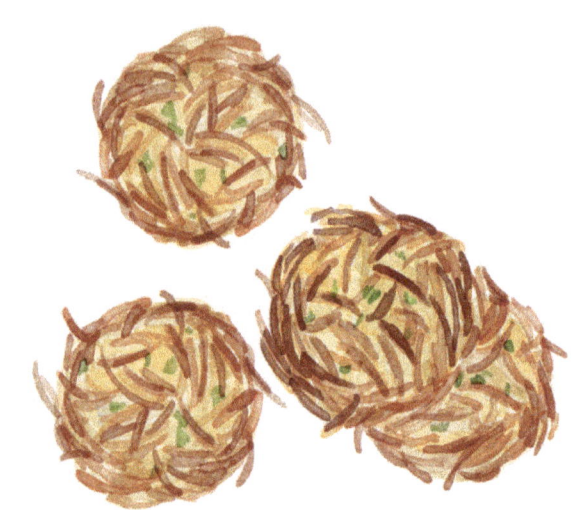

Grate the potatoes and onion using a food processor.
Transfer to a clean dish towel, squeeze, wringing out as much of the liquid as possible.
Transfer the mixture to a large bowl and add the eggs, sprinkle with potato
starch, salt, and pepper to the bowl; mix well.
Scoop out heaping tablespoons of mixture, try to squeeze as much moisture out before placing onto a baking pan lined with parchment paper, use the back of a spoon to gently flatten.
Brush the tops of the latkes with some of the softened ghee.

Bake for 10-12 minutes, flip (brush a little more ghee) and repeat.

Serve with Homemade Applesauce for tradition or organic sour cream for a modern twist with chopped chives.

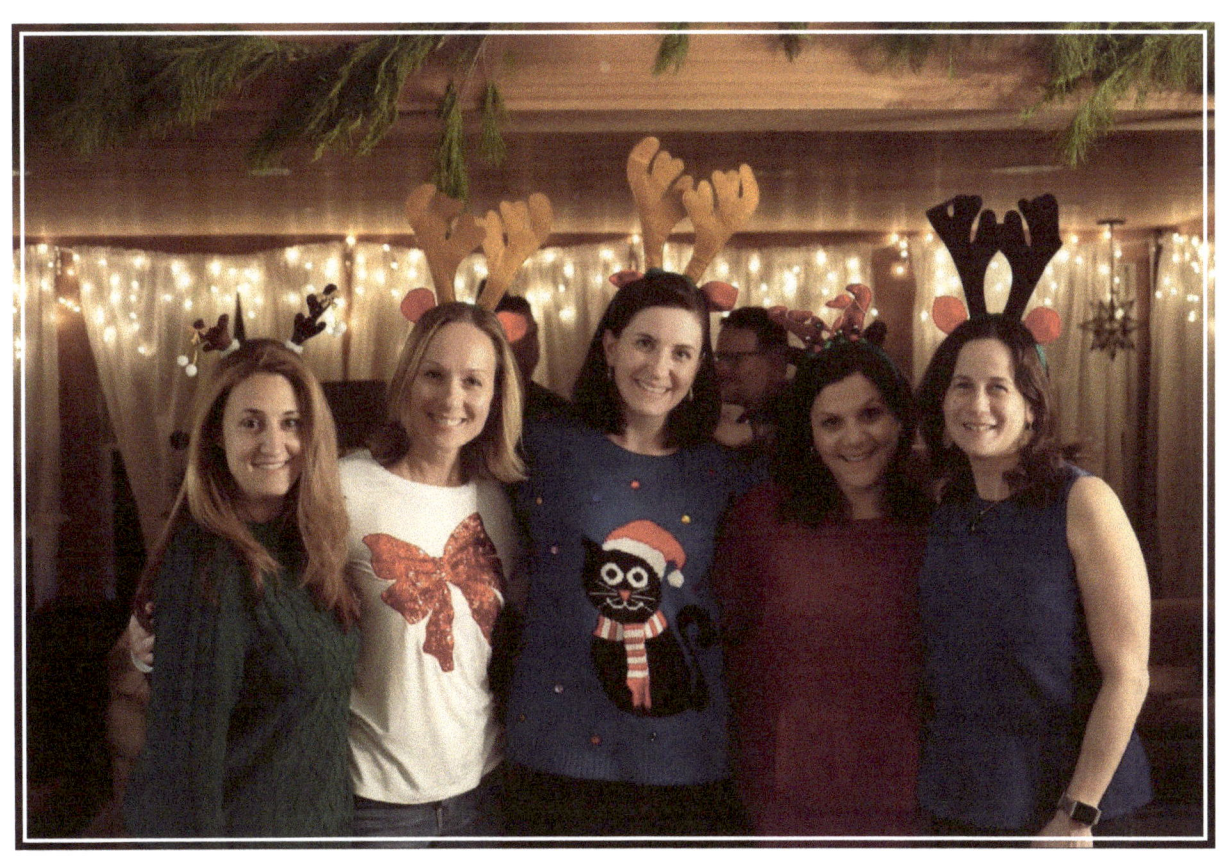

We gather for the most anticipated night of the year

BAKED PLANTAINS

This makes a special side dish for our Roasted Lemon Chicken and Yellow Rice.

- ✓ 2-4 Ripe Plantains
- ✓ Avocado Oil

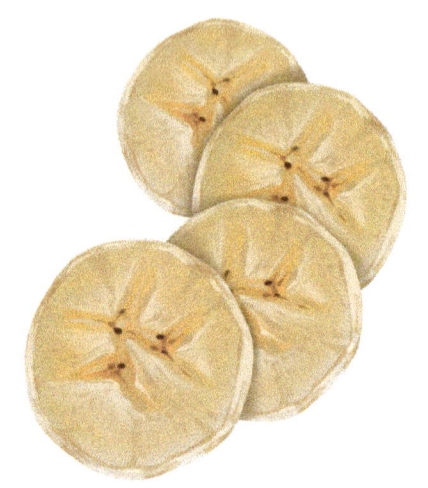

Peel and slice Plantains on a diagonal about ½-¾" thick.

Lightly oil a parchment lined baking sheet and place individual slices down without overlapping. In a 350°F oven, bake for 20 minutes, turn over and bake another 10-20 minutes.

They should be golden brown on the outside and still soft inside.

BAKING IS FUN, add SOMETHING SWEET

ANTIOXIDANT TRUFFLES

This is the Land of Nutrition Cornerstone recipe, always a hit, and always a healthy alternative to a sweet treat, each ingredient offers antioxidants to keep you feeling your best.

INGREDIENTS

- ✓ 1 Cup Organic Pitted Dates (soak in water for 30 min)
- ✓ 1/4 cup Unsweetened Shredded Coconut
- ✓ 1/4 cup Cacao Powder
- ✓ 2T chia seeds
- ✓ 2T ground flax seed (or more)
- ✓ 1T coconut oil melted
- ✓ 1-2 tsp vanilla extract
- ✓ pinch sea salt
- ✓ 1-2 Tbsp Cacao Nibs or Mini Chocolate chips (optional)

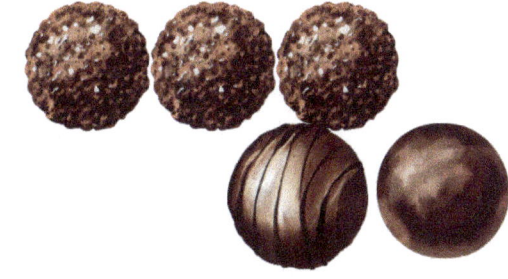

Drain Dates and add to a food processor with additional ingredients, Process until well combined, forming into a mixed large ball.

Roll into Tablespoon sizes, I like to use a measuring spoon and tiny spatula to make equal size mounds, then roll into balls. These keep in the fridge for a week or in the freezer for 3 months, if they last that long!

FOOL PROOF IRISH SODA BREAD

For St. Patrick's Day, everyone is Irish - ALL (well, a lot, even the true Irish ones) of my friends ask me for this recipe and text/call send pics on St Patty's day thinking of me because this is really the BEST Irish Soda bread ever!!! I've made upwards of 8-10 per year for Bill to take to clients and for neighbors, family and friends. It's the first thing to go at our annual, one time a year, corned beef and Guinness party. You should know by now, health is more than just what's on your plate, and this is one of life's little indulgences. The key is, as always, to use the highest quality ingredients you can find.
Enjoy!

INGREDIENTS
(MAKES 2 ROUND IRISH SODA BREADS)

- 5 cups all-purpose unbleached flour, sifted if you want
- 3/4 cup sugar
- 2 teaspoons baking powder
- 1 1/2 teaspoons salt
- 1 teaspoon baking soda
- 1/4 pound (1 stick) butter at room temperature
- 2 1/2 cups mixed light and dark raisins, soaked in water for 15 to 20 minutes and drained
- 2-3 tablespoons caraway seeds (or omit all together)
- 2 1/2 cups buttermilk
- 1 large egg, slightly beaten

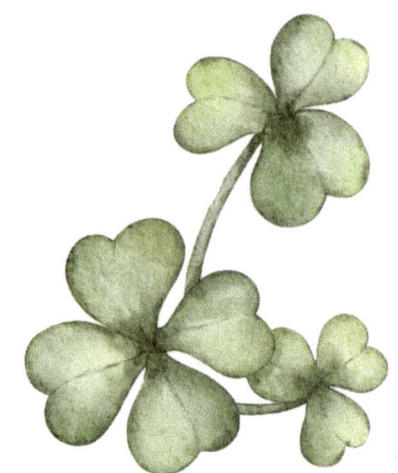

Preheat the oven to 350ºF. Generously butter 2 round cake pans.
Stir together the flour, sugar, baking powder, salt, and baking soda. Cut in the butter and mix very thoroughly with your hands until it gets grainy.
Stir in raisins and caraway seeds.
Beat the egg and buttermilk in a bowl and then add to the flour mixture. Stir until well moistened. Pour dough into the two round buttered pans.
Bake for 1 hour. Test with a toothpick for doneness. Cool in the pans for a few minutes then transfer to a wire rack to cool. Test slice a warm piece with Kerrygold grass fed butter.
Sláinte.

COCONUT MACAROONS

I LOVE COCONUT and these Macaroons are not only good for you, a healthy serving of good fats from the coconut meat and no sugar, but taste amazing. You will never miss the sugar or artificial additives from store bought. Eat them fast or store them in the freezer!

INGREDIENTS

- ✓ 1 ¼ Cups of Unsweetened Shredded Coconut
- ✓ ¾ cups of Blanched Almond Flour
- ✓ 3 Tbsp Organic Virgin Coconut Oil
- ✓ ¼ cup of 100% Maple Syrup
- ✓ 2 Egg Whites
- ✓ (Optional add mini chocolate chips, I love the brand Enjoy Life)

Preheat your oven to 350°F. Add all ingredients to a Food Processor and pulse until well combined and resembles a thick batter. Add another tablespoon or 2 of shredded coconut after blending and add mini chips after blending as well.
Scoop 1 Tbsp ball onto a parchment lined cookie sheet.
Bake for 12-14 minutes. Remove immediately to avoid burnt bottoms.
Enjoy!!

Tip: Putting a sheet of Aluminum Foil on the bottom rack of your oven can help avoid burnt bottoms.

LAND OF NUTRITION GRANOLA

DRY INGREDIENTS:

- ✓ 3C Pumpkin Seeds
- ✓ 1.5 C Sunflower Seeds
- ✓ 1 C Sliced Almonds
- ✓ 1/2 C Flax Seeds (whole) or try Hemp Seeds
- ✓ 3T Chia Seeds
- ✓ 1t Cinnamon
- ✓ 1t Cardamom
- ✓ 1/2t Sea Salt

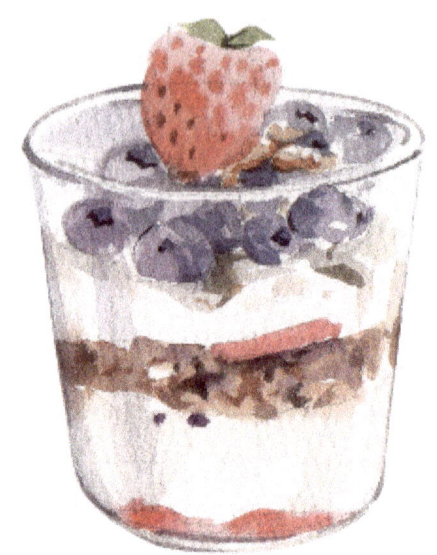

WET INGREDIENTS:

- ✓ 1/3 C melted coconut oil or Avocado Oil
- ✓ 2/3 C Maple Syrup
- ✓ 1t Vanilla Extract

Mix dry ingredients in a large bowl. (If you like oats in your granola, this recipe is flexible and customizable to your liking – just add Oats). Go ahead, play with the ratios of seeds and nuts, try Buckwheat Groats, Pistachio Nutmeat or Hemp Seeds: Dry Ingredients should total 6 Cups. Whisk oil, maple syrup and vanilla and pour over dry ingredients.
Mix well. Line Baking Sheet with Parchment paper, spread mixture evenly.
Bake at 350°F for 25-30 min, until golden.
Remove from the oven, the mixture will harden after a few minutes.

Tip: Putting a sheet of Aluminum Foil on the bottom rack of your oven can help avoid burnt bottoms.

Hot tip: I find that the bottom layer keeps cooking on the hot pan, so I often transfer the parchment with granola on top to my cool countertop to let it harden.
Store in an airtight container for up to a week (if it lasts that long).
Serve over Organic Greek Yogurt, as a snack or toss a few Tablespoons of it over your salad for a sweet crunch.

If you like oats in your granola, this recipe is flexible and customizable to your liking – just add Oats. Go ahead, play with the ratios of seeds and nuts, try Buckwheat Groats, Pistachio Nutmeat or Hemp Seeds: Dry Ingredients should total 6 Cups.

Try my daughter, Olivia's, favorite ratios: 3 Cups Organic Gluten Free Oats, 1 Cup Organic Sprouted Pumpkin seeds, 1 cup sliced almonds, ½ cup Sunflower seeds, ½ cup mix of Organic Whole Flax Seeds, Hemp seeds and Chia seeds.

Space to write your favorite ratios here:

BERRY NICE BOARD

This is a great alternative to standard brownie, cake and cookie desserts and will leave you feeling much better too:

Tray of Berries add dark Chocolate (Like a cheese platter but better)

Think:
- ✓ Strawberries
- ✓ Blueberries
- ✓ Raspberries
- ✓ Blackberries
- ✓ Pumpkin Seeds, almonds
- ✓ Shaved Coconut pieces
- ✓ Good Quality Dark Chocolate Bar broken into pieces

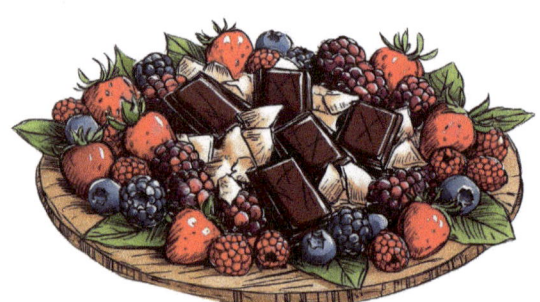

Put Vitamin L (love) in designing a beautiful dessert platter!

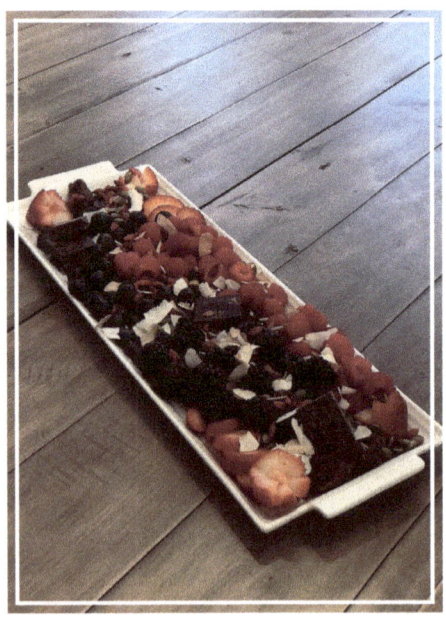

SWEET POTATO BROWNIES

The sweet potato adds a beautiful sweetness to this sugar free brownie. This recipe combines the nutrient-rich sweet potatoes packed with fiber and vitamins, healthy fats and protein from almond butter and almond flour, antioxidant-rich cacao, and natural sweetness from pure maple syrup, making a wholesome, satisfying treat.

INGREDIENTS

- ¾ cup Sweet Potato (Roast 2 Sweet Potatoes until soft, around 40 minutes, scoop the insides)
- 3/4 cup Organic Almond Butter
- 1/2 cup Cacao Powder
- 1/2 cup 100% Pure Maple Syrup
- 1/4 cup Almond Flour
- 1/4 cup mini chocolate chips

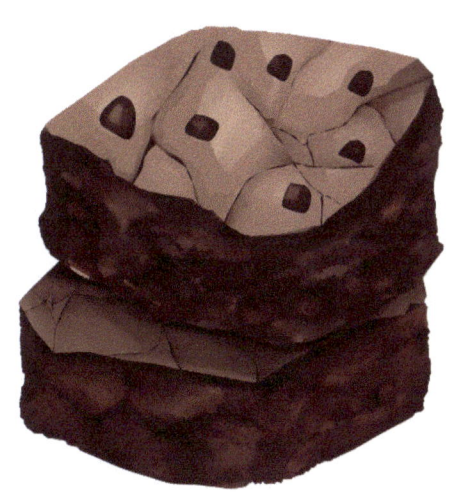

Mix all ingredients until well blended.
Bake 350°F for 45 minutes in a 9x9 parchment lined baking dish.
Let cool completely and cut into 16 even squares.

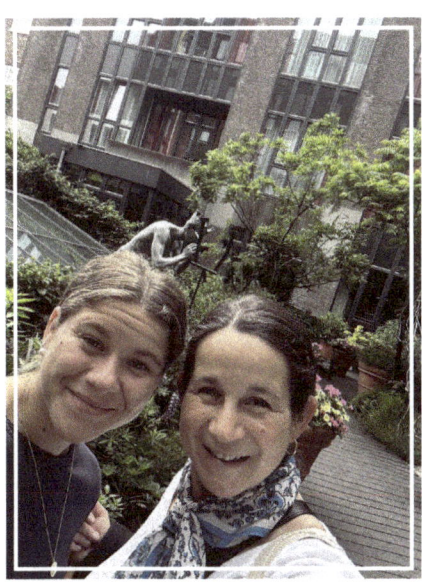
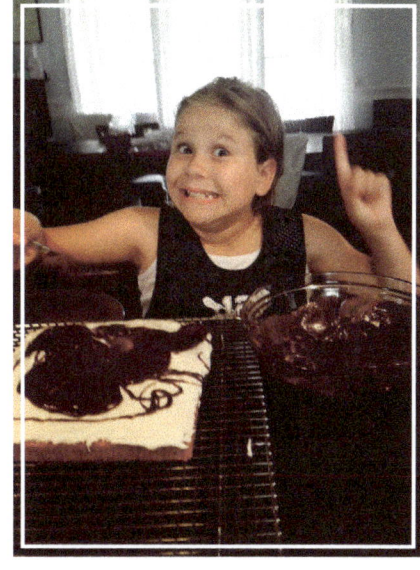

HEART HEALTHY LINZER TARTS WITH CHIA SEED JAM

Linzer Tarts are my favorite! Been giving myself some love with experimenting in the kitchen! The result is a healthy version of a Valentine's Day classic!! These cookies, on their own, are yummy. But paired with raspberry chia seed jam, they are something to fall in love with!

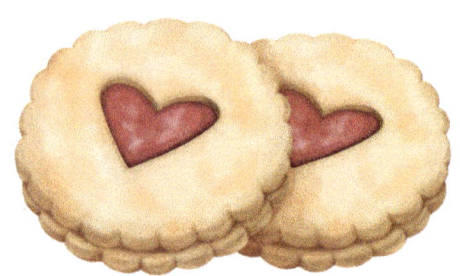

First, make Chia seed jam filling
(This can also be used as a yogurt topping, spread for toast or a yummy teaspoon in your matcha tea, another nutrient powerhouse to try.)

In a small sauce pot add:
- ✓ 1 1/2 Cups of frozen raspberries (or strawberries)
- ✓ 2 Tablespoons of honey
- ✓ 2 Tbsp Chia Seeds and a squeeze of fresh lemon juice

Simmer for about 10 minutes. Be careful not to burn bottom by stirring often, learn from my experience. Let cool to room temperature and refrigerate once cool.

Make the cookies!
- ✓ Set aside 2 room temperature organic eggs from free range chickens and
- ✓ ½ Cup melted coconut oil.

Whisk together dry ingredients:
- ✓ 1 1/4 Cup of Almond Flour
- ✓ 1/4 cup coconut flour
- ✓ 1/2 cup coconut sugar
- ✓ 1tsp baking powder
- ✓ 1/2 tsp baking soda
- ✓ 1/2t cinnamon

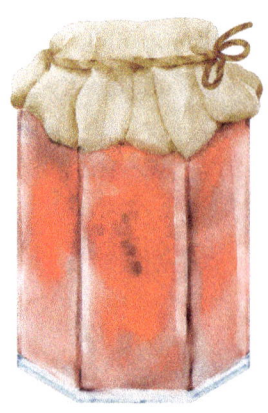

- ✓ 1/4t nutmeg
- ✓ pinch of sea salt

Use a hand mixer or food processor to whisk 2 organic eggs for 30 seconds, add coconut oil, then pulse in dry ingredients until it comes together into dough. If it's too dry, you can add a splash of coconut milk (or water).

Drop dough on parchment paper, cover with another piece of parchment paper, refrigerate for 20-30 minutes - roll out to 1/4".

Cut with cookie cutters of choice. I love hearts.

Bake on a parchment lined cookie sheet for 10 minutes at 350°F.

Cool immediately on wire racks.

Assemble cookies by spreading jam on the bottom cookie and you can lightly dust the top with a mix of 1/2 Coconut Flour/1/2 Coconut sugar.

Store in an airtight container in the fridge for a few days.

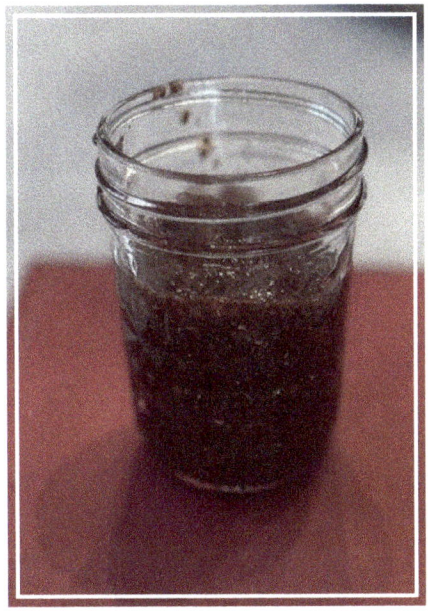
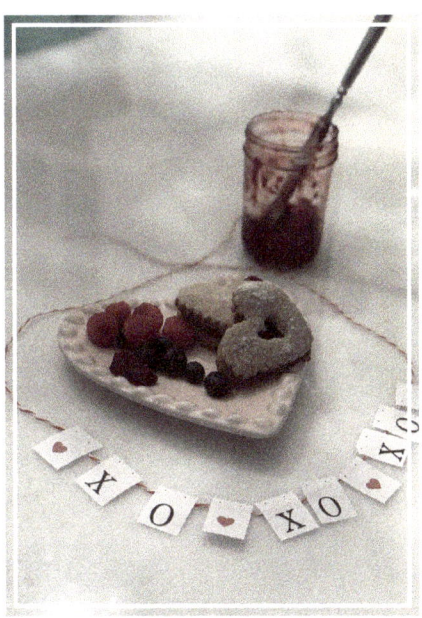

ZUCCHINI MUFFINS

Zucchini is plentiful come summertime and amazing for your health. Loaded with vitamin C, for your anti-aging and antioxidant needs, lowers blood sugar levels, great source of fiber, great for heart health, improves digestion, supports adrenal glands, reduces stress the list goes on!! Try this now for great energy: blend it with cucumber, frozen pineapple, avocado, mint!
When you have an abundance, try this delicious muffin recipe:

DRY INGREDIENTS

- ✓ 2 cups Organic All Purpose flour, or try Einkorn Flour, whole wheat flour, or a mix added to 2C)
- ✓ 1 cup Almond flour (or whole wheat flour)
- ✓ 2 Tbsp Ground Flax Meal
- ✓ 1/2 tsp baking powder
- ✓ 1 tsp baking soda
- ✓ 1 tsp salt
- ✓ 3 tsp cinnamon

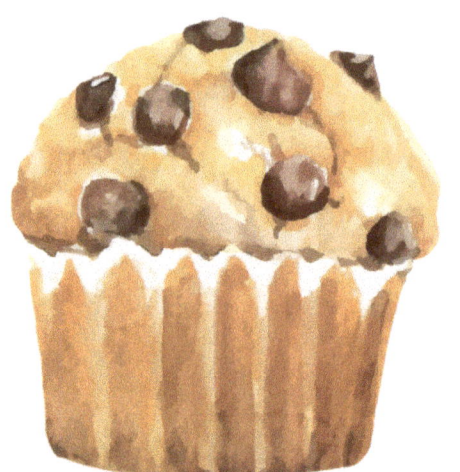

MIX WET INGREDIENTS

- ✓ 4 Large eggs - Beat these first then slowly add
- ✓ 1 cup EVOO
- ✓ 1 Cup Coconut sugar
- ✓ 1 tsp vanilla extract

COMBINE AND FOLD IN:

- ✓ 4 cups zucchini, grated and moisture squeezed out - Really Squeeze it out
- ✓ 1/2 cup mini chocolate chips

PREHEAT OVEN TO 350°F.

Whisk the dry ingredients together in a large bowl. In a separate medium bowl, beat eggs until foamy, Add vanilla extract, coconut sugar, mix well, then drizzle 1 cup olive oil while whisking.

Pour wet ingredients into the large bowl and mix well with the dry, then fold in shredded zucchini and chocolate chips.

Makes 24 muffins. Or make a loaf! It may take a little longer, you will know it's done when you can insert a toothpick and it comes out dry Bake for 25-30 min. Set to cool on wire rack.

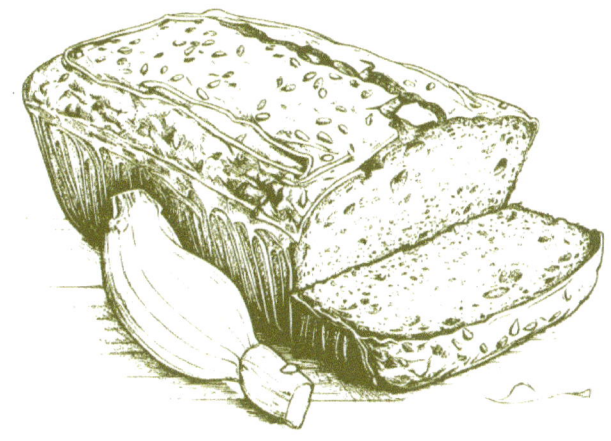

LARA'S ALMOND BUTTER CHUNKS

Always in my freezer, these chunks are packed with protein, healthy fats, fiber, antioxidants, and natural sweetness, supporting muscle repair, heart health, and sustained energy.

- ✓ 2 cups or One 16 oz jar of No Salt Added ALMOND BUTTER, crunchy or smooth
- ✓ 1 Cup Chocolate Protein Powder of your choice
- ✓ 1 Cup Sunflower seeds
- ✓ 1 Cup Sliced Almonds
- ✓ ¼ cup Ground Flax meal
- ✓ ½-3/4 cup of 100% pure Maple syrup
- ✓ 1/4-1/2 cup Chocolate Chips

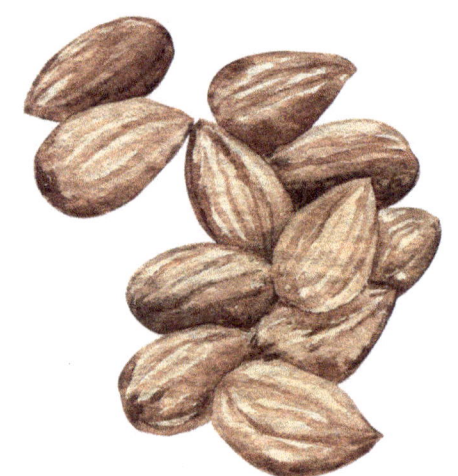

Add each of the above ingredients to a large bowl, mixing well after each ingredient.
Line a rectangle baking pan with parchment paper. Spread mixture evenly in pan top with another sheet parchment spread out to edges, smooth (I use a smaller square baking pan on top to smooth it out.)
Freeze for an hour or more. Cut into 1" squares, keep in the freezer and eat when you need a healthy snack and boost of energy.

TAHINI SQUARES

This no bake recipe was inspired by a very expensive brand's treat - nailed it here Tahini is a creamy paste made from ground sesame seeds, and it's good for you because it's rich in healthy fats, plant-based protein, fiber, and important nutrients like calcium, magnesium, and antioxidants that support heart health, bone strength, and overall wellness. A truly nourishing and satisfying snack or dessert.

Step 1
1 Cup Tahini
¼ cup 100% pure Maple Syrup
1 Cup Almond Flour
1 tsp Vanilla Extract
Pinch sea salt
½ c mini chocolate chips (we love the brand Enjoy Life mini chips)
Mix all ingredients and press into a parchment lined 8x8 square pan.

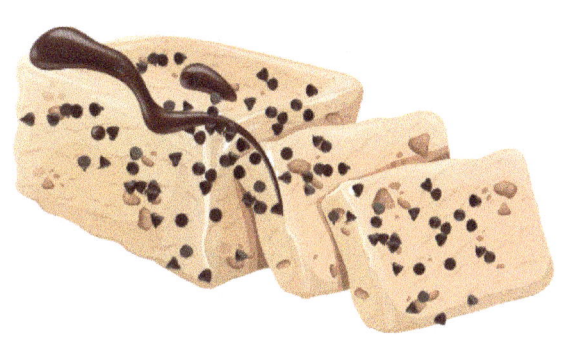

Step 2
Melt 1 Cup Chocolate Chips (we love Enjoy Life Chocolate Chunks)
1 Tbsp Coconut Oil
Pour over tahini mix, sprinkle flaky sea salt (we love Maldon).
Freeze for 1 hour to harden, cut into squares and keep in the freezer.

BANANA BREAD

When selecting recipes for this book, I choose recipes that I make most often or most requested by friends and family. The key is, as always, to use the highest quality ingredients you can find. This banana bread is a standard in our house for sure. When bananas turn soft, we whip this up.

You can also freeze the soft bananas to use another time. Blend them up on their own to make "nice cream," an ice cream consistency, a sweet treat without all the added sugar or dairy!

INGREDIENTS

- [x] 1 1/2 cups AP flour or Whole Wheat Flour
- [x] 1 1/2 teaspoons baking powder
- [x] 1/2 teaspoon baking soda
- [x] 1/2 teaspoon sea salt
- [x] 1 teaspoon ground cinnamon
- [x] 1/2 cup organic sugar
- [x] 2 Eggs from free range, organic fed chickens
- [x] 1/2 cup greek yogurt
- [x] 1 tsp vanilla extract
- [x] 2 tablespoons butter, melted
- [x] 3 large ripe bananas
- [x] 1/2 cup mini chocolate chips (optional)

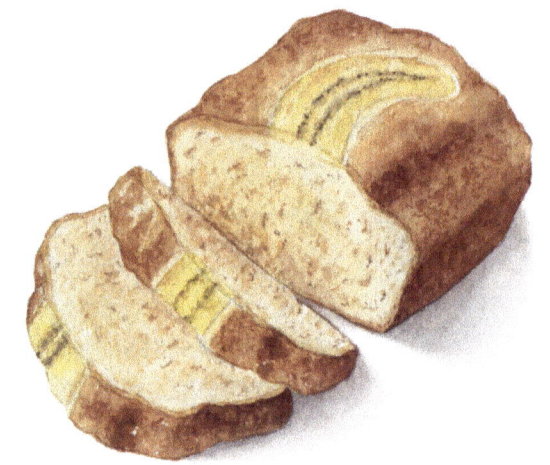

Preheat oven to 350°F, Line a 9X5 loaf pan with parchment paper.
In a medium bowl, combine dry ingredients: flour, baking powder, baking soda, salt, and cinnamon.
In a large bowl, with an electric mixer, beat sugar and egg. Blend in yogurt, vanilla extract and butter.
Mash bananas with a fork and stir into yogurt mixture. Combine dry and wet ingredients well. Then fold in chocolate chips. Pour into the prepared pan.
Bake for 50 minutes - until a toothpick inserted in the middle comes out clean.
Cool pan on a wire rack.

ELIXIRS

Besides Herbal Tea, I often use these tonics in addition to my daily hydration.

MAGIC MORNING TONIC

Ginger, turmeric, and honey make a powerhouse mix — ginger aids digestion and eases inflammation, turmeric's curcumin fights oxidative stress and supports joint health, and raw honey offers antioxidants, soothes the throat, and boosts immunity. Together, they're a warming, healing blend for overall vitality.

IN A SMALL JAR ADD:

- ✓ 1/2 C local raw Honey
- ✓ 2t Ground Turmeric
- ✓ 2t Ground Ginger
- ✓ A good pinch of black pepper (helps the turmeric absorb).

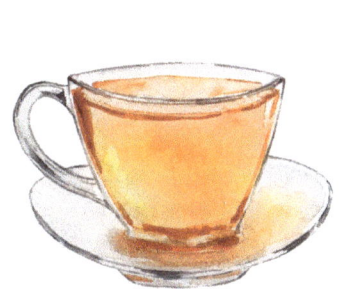
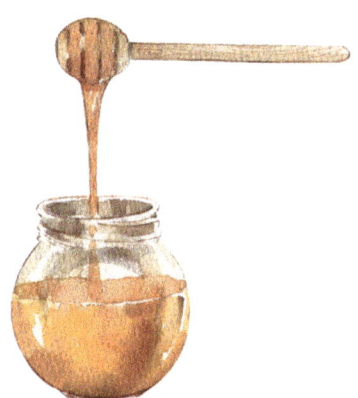

Keep in a dark cabinet. Add a teaspoon to warm water to start your morning in a fresh way. You can also add the juice from half a lemon to kick start your liver and get ready for the amazing work it does for you and your digestion, without you even knowing it - think of how amazing our bodies truly are.

I usually take this to the back door and step outside or window (if you live in an apartment), drink in the golden drink and feel the natural sunlight on your skin. There you go, another boost of Vitamin D. And don't forget the L, for love.

NIGHT TIME CHERRY JUICE MOCKTAIL

This is my "I'm making dinner, tired of water," drink that is really beneficial for sleep in more ways than one. The tart cherry juice provides naturally occurring tryptophan (an amino acid that helps the body produce melatonin, which helps to calm inflammation, ease muscle tension, and quiet the day's mental noise, supporting deeper rest). Ashwagandha, an adaptogen, can help regulate our hormones and reduce anxiety.

- ✓ 6oz Water
- ✓ 2 oz Unsweetened Tart Cherry Juice
- ✓ Juice from half lime squeezed
- ✓ Magnesium powder and/or drop of Ashwagandha

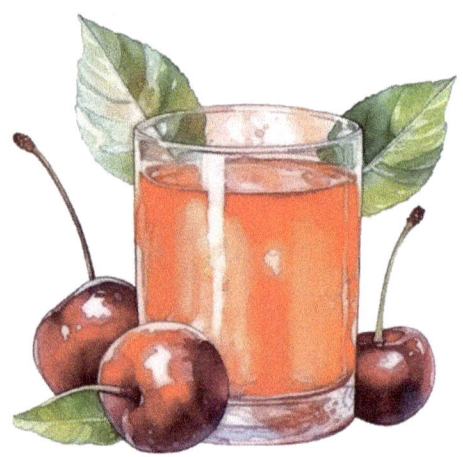

THANKSGIVING MENU

Hosting this non-denominational holiday has become second nature with this healthy and easy menu

Crudités Appetizer
Use farm fresh veggies: Carrots, broccoli (lightly steamed or raw), cauliflower, various radishes (french, watermelon, white salad), endive, peppers. Get creative. Lay cut veggies on a cabbage leaf, assort by rainbow, serve with hummus or this homemade salad dressing as dip:
Land of Nutrition House Salad Dressing: 1/4 cup Good Extra Virgin Olive Oil, 1/4 cup White Balsamic Vinegar, 1 tsp Dijon mustard, Pinch of sea salt, Put all in a jar and shake.
One of my favorite indulgences is a cheese board. However, I have learned to add healthier options make me feel so much better inside: Kalamata Olives, Pumpkin Seeds, Goji Berries, sliced radishes

SIDE DISHES
Classic Mashed Potatoes
Russet Potatoes make the best mash! Cook potatoes in boiling, salted water for 20 minutes or until tender. Drain well. Place in a crockpot to keep warm while all else goes on in the kitchen. Mash with 8oz Grass Fed Butter and S&P to taste. BONUS: Serve these with caramelized onions.

Brussel Sprouts with Nitrate free Bacon
Brussel Sprouts are worth all of the effort! Par Boil brussel sprouts a day before to save time on the big day. Cut bacon into ½" pieces and cook on medium-low heat in a saute pan, once crispy, add brussel sprouts and cook for about 7 more minutes, I like to stir often, loosening the layers of the sprouts.

Roasted Carrots with Thyme
8-10 local organic colored carrots and scrub with veggie brush, don't peel! Slice on the diagonal to 2" pieces. Lay on baking pan, drizzle 2 Tbsp EVOO and 1T Dried thyme, or fresh if you have it. Bake at 350°F for 15-20 min.

Homemade Sourdough and Whole Wheat Stuffing

We don't actually stuff the bird but make this on the side in a casserole dish..

Start by forcing 2 loaves of bread stale by laying them on a baking tray overnight on the counter, toast them lightly on Thanksgiving morning. Melt 2 sticks of unsalted butter and saute a mirepoix (diced carrots, onion and celery). Cut bread into small pieces and put in a large bowl. Pour the softened veggies and butter over the diced bread, add salt pepper, garlic powder and chopped parsley, and about 2 cups of broth. Spread in a baking dish and bake at 350°F covered with foil for 40 minutes then uncover and bake for another 10 minutes.

THE BIRD

TURKEY 1.5lb per person

Stuff the bird with carrots, onions and celery – make "dressing" aka Stuffing in a baking dish

Roast the bird breast side down for the first few hours on a wire rack in a baking pan.

Comes out perfect every time.

Leaving it to the expert (see link) to explain, don't over complicate it.
https://www.marthastewart.com/1164831/upside-down-turkey

DESSERT

In any baking dish: Slice some apples, sprinkle some cinnamon, lemon juice, top with oats, coconut sugar and some more cinnamon, Bake in a 350°F oven for 20-25 minutes.

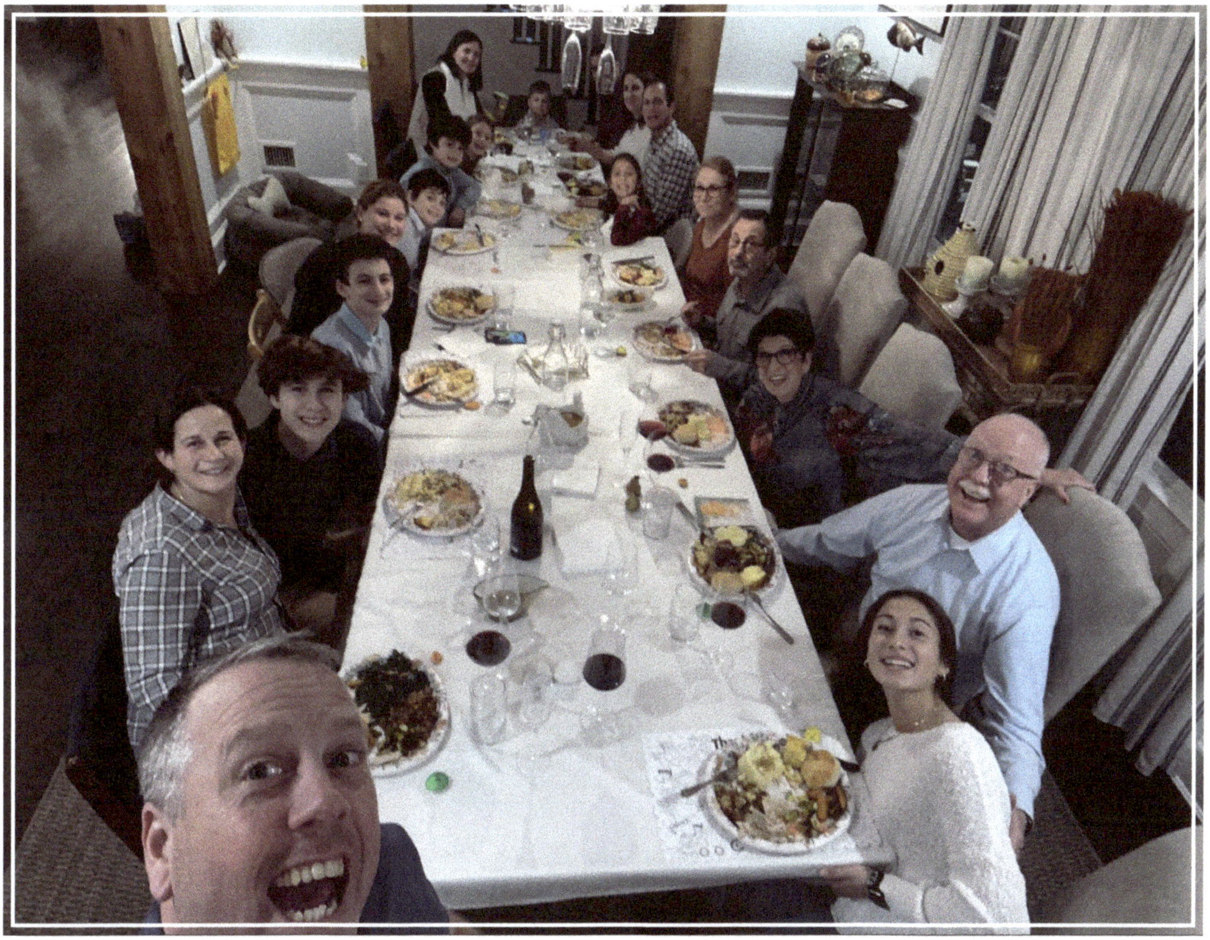

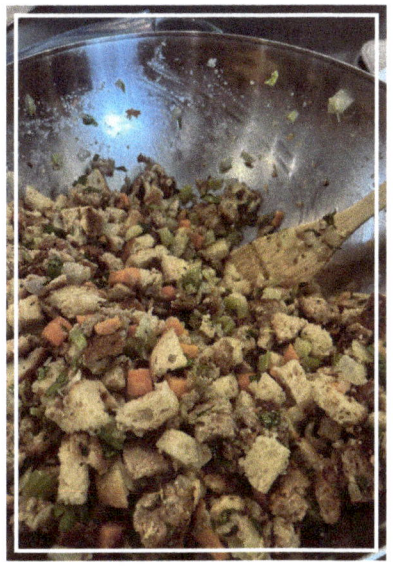
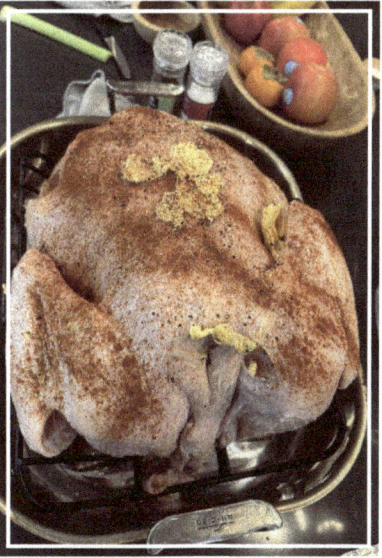
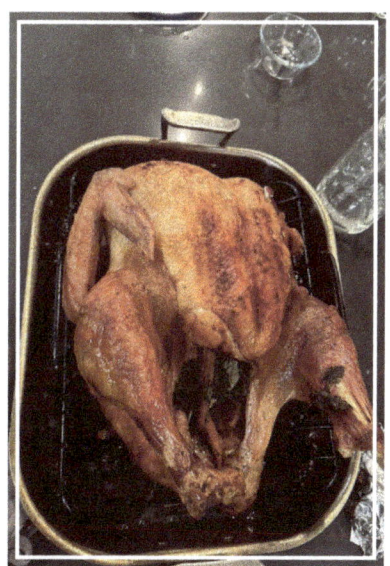

THANKSGIVING MENU

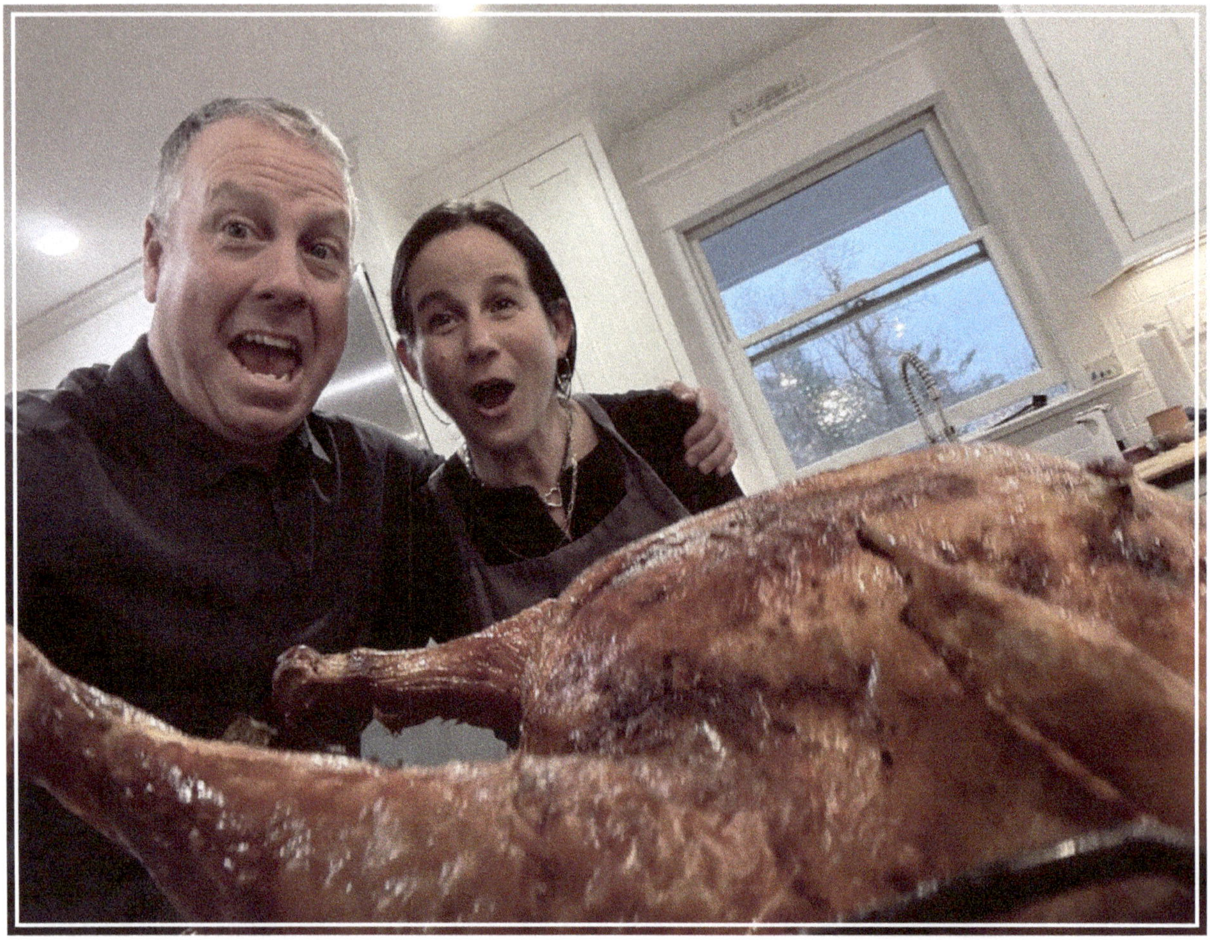

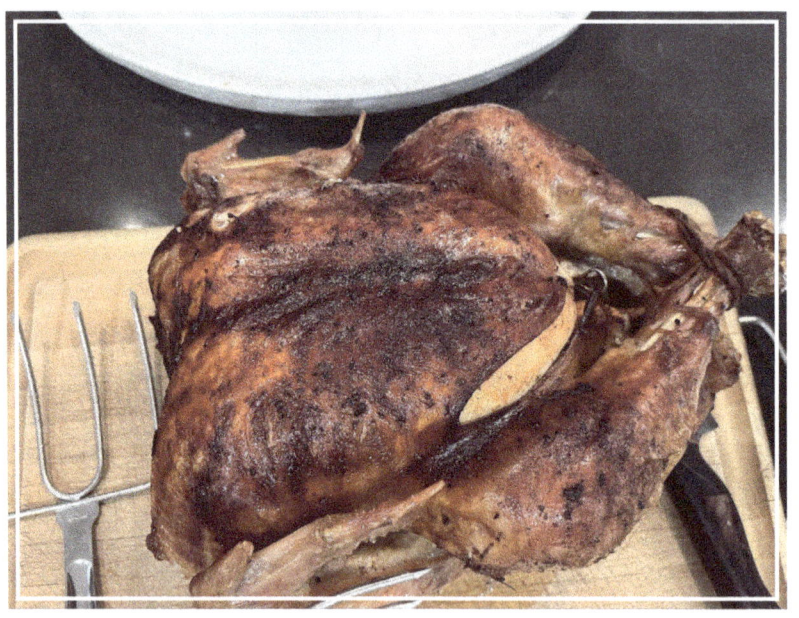

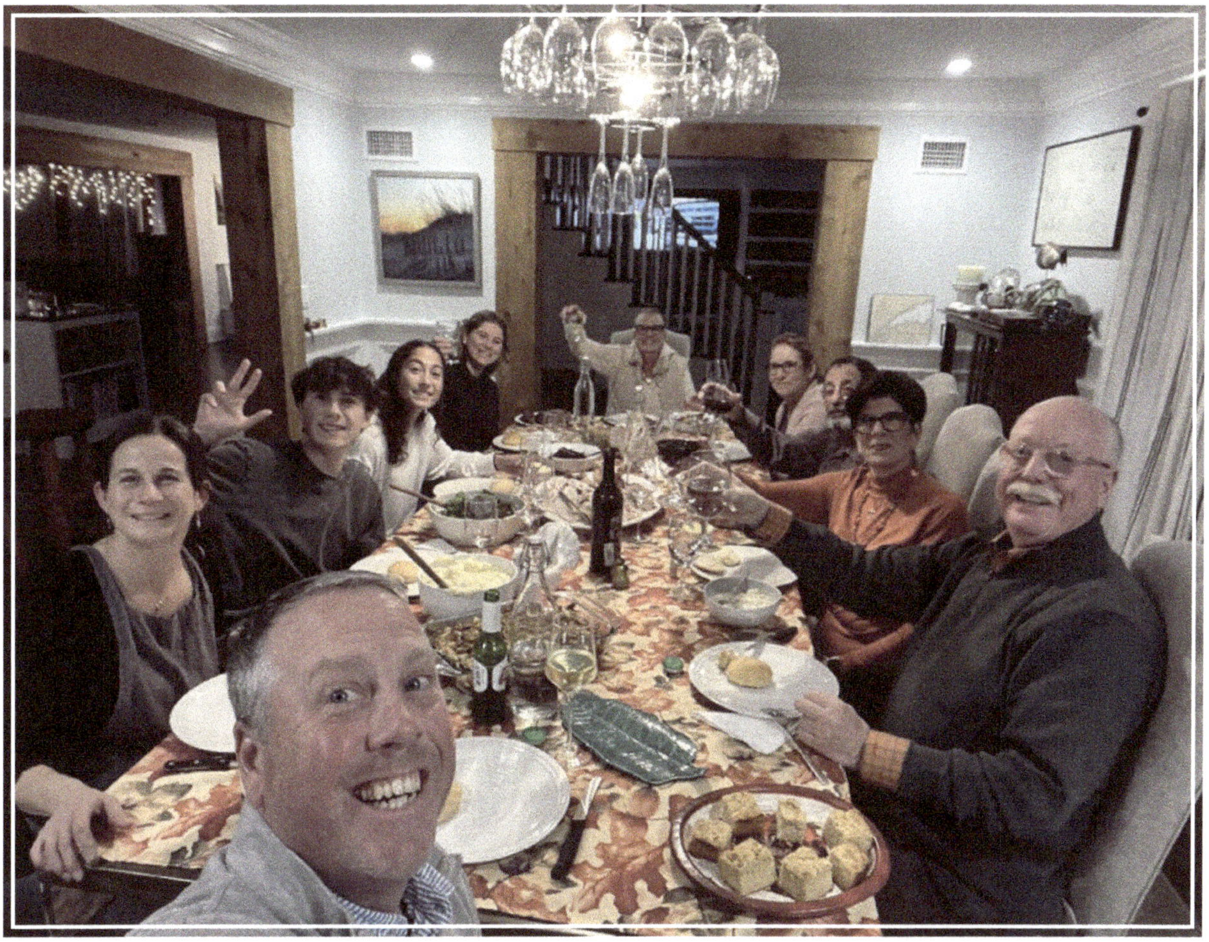

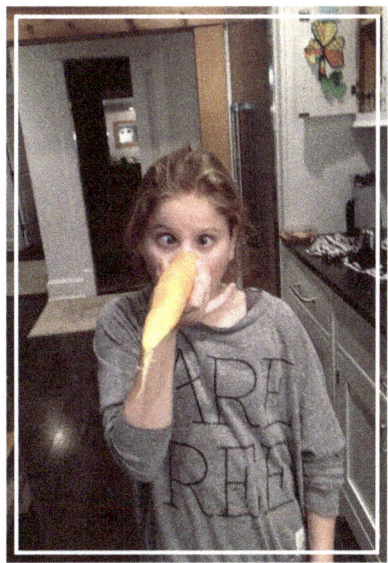
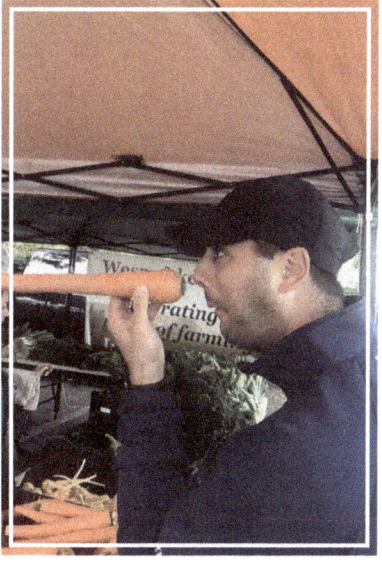

roots are fun

THANKSGIVING MENU

Seasonal Hits (when in doubt, check this out)

SPRING

- ✓ St Patrick's Day Irish Soda Bread
- ✓ Mother's Day Spring Vegetable Frittata with Mixed Greens Salad
- ✓ Easter Baby Lamb Chops Dry-ish Marinade
- ✓ Passover Coconut Macaroons

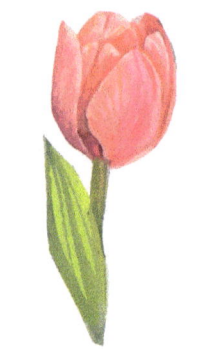

SUMMER CLASSICS

- ✓ Grilled grass fed steaks, Green beans, Chimichurri Green Sauce
- ✓ Grass Fed Beef Burgers and Hot Dogs, homemade Saurkraut
- ✓ Summer Salad
- ✓ Skirt Steak Marinade with Chimichurri
- ✓ Gazpacho Chilled Soup
- ✓ Zucchini Muffins

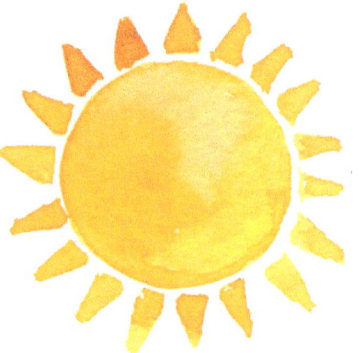

AUTUMN

- ✓ Butternut Squash Soup
- ✓ Rosh Hashanah Uncle Stu's Chicken Noodle Soup
- ✓ Stripe-Tober aka Cape Cod Cod
- ✓ Chilli
- ✓ Thanksgiving Menu

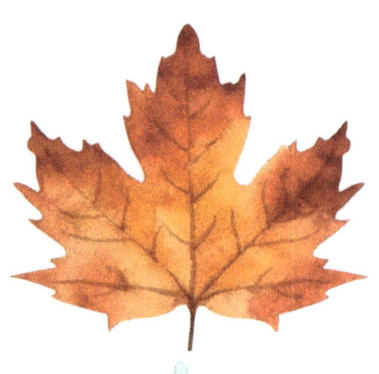

WINTER

- ✓ Ramen Radish Noodle Soup
- ✓ Sauerkraut
- ✓ TNT Tacos
- ✓ Hanukkah Latkes and homemade applesauce
- ✓ Christmas Salad and go to meal

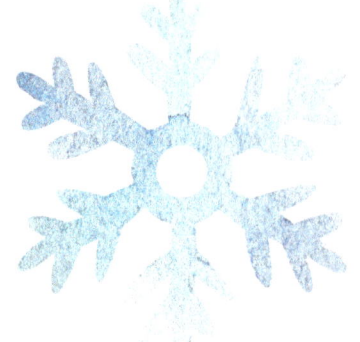

Reference Guide

For more on the impact of freezing and toasting on the glycaemic response of white bread, see: Burton, P. Lightowler, H. J., & Henry, C. J. K. (2008).

The impact of freezing and toasting on the glycaemic response of white bread
https://pmc.ncbi.nlm.nih.gov/articles/PMC3249911

On the connection between gluten, inflammation, and neurodegeneration, see: Cardona, F., Andrés-Lacueva, C., Tulipani, S., Tinahones, F. J., & Queipo-Ortuño, M. I. (2022).

Gluten, Inflammation, and Neurodegeneration
https://pmc.ncbi.nlm.nih.gov/articles/PMC3614697/

Nutritional characteristics of Parmesean Reggiano
https://www.parmigianoreggiano.com/product-guide-nutritional-characteristics

Free radicals, antioxidants and functional foods: Impact on human health
https://pmc.ncbi.nlm.nih.gov/articles/PMC3249911

Free Radicals, Antioxidants in Disease and Health
https://pmc.ncbi.nlm.nih.gov/articles/PMC3614697/

Philip A, White ND. Gluten, Inflammation, and Neurodegeneration. Am J Lifestyle Med. 2022 Jan 11;16(1):32-35. doi: 10.1177/15598276211049345. PMID: 35185424; PMCID: PMC8848113.
https://pmc.ncbi.nlm.nih.gov/articles/PMC8848113/

The Dirty Dozen™
https://www.ewg.org/foodnews/dirty-dozen.php

The Clean Fifteen™
https://www.ewg.org/foodnews/clean-fifteen.php

Uncovering How Microbes in the Soil Influence Our Health and Our Food
https://www.washingtonpost.com/science/uncovering-how-microbes-in-the-soil-influence-our-health-and-our-food/2019/09/27/81634f54-a4ba-11e9-bd56-eac6bb02d01d_story.html

Food additive emulsifiers and cancer risk: Results from the French prospective NutriNet-Santé cohort.
https://journals.plos.org/plosmedicine/article?id=10.1371/journal.pmed.1004338

What is Maltodextrin?
https://www.webmd.com/diet/what-is-maltodextrin#1-2

Is Maltodextrin Safe?
https://www.medicalnewstoday.com/articles/322426#safety-and-side-effects

Mindfulness & Compassion Practices

Metta Institute.
https://www.mettainstitute.org/

Salzberg S. Loving-kindness meditation. Mindful Magazine.
https://www.mindful.org/loving-kindness-meditation-with-sharon-salzberg/

Genetically Modified Foods & Agriculture

Genetically modified rice could be key to tackling food shortages caused by climate change. PreventionWeb.
https://www.preventionweb.net/news/genetically-modified-rice-could-be-key-tackling-food-shortages-caused-climate-change

Séralini GE, Cellier D, de Vendomois JS. New analysis of a rat feeding study with a genetically modified maize reveals signs of hepatorenal toxicity. Archives of Environmental Contamination and Toxicology, 2007; 52(4):596-602. doi:10.1007/s00244-006-0149-5

Non-GMO corn outperforms GM corn in several US states. Biosafety Information Centre.
https://biosafety-info.net/articles/assessment-impacts/socioeconomic/non-gmo-corn-outperforms-gm-corn-in-several-us-states

GM soybean oil damages liver and kidneys. GMWatch.
https://www.gmwatch.org/en/106-news/latest-news/20467-gm-soybean-oil-damages-liver-and-kidneys

Kiliç A, Akay MT. A three generation study with genetically modified Bt corn in rats: Biochemical and histopathological investigation. Food and Chemical Toxicology, 2008; 46(3):1164-70. doi:10.1016/j.fct.2007.11.016

Use of genetically modified organism (GMO)-containing food products in children. Pediatrics, 2024; 153(1): e2023064774. doi:10.1542/peds.2023-064774

Food Additives & Ingredients

The Dirty Dozen: BHA and BHT. David Suzuki Foundation.
https://davidsuzuki.org/living-green/dirty-dozen-bha-bht/

Chazelas E, et al. Food additive emulsifiers and cancer risk: Results from the French prospective NutriNet-Santé cohort. PLOS Medicine, 2024; 21(2): e1004338.
https://journals.plos.org/plosmedicine/article?id=10.1371/journal.pmed.1004338

Nutrition & Health

Fats and cholesterol. Harvard T.H. Chan School of Public Health – The Nutrition Source.
https://nutritionsource.hsph.harvard.edu/what-should-you-eat/fats-and-cholesterol/

Toxicology of food dyes. PubMed.
https://pubmed.ncbi.nlm.nih.gov/23026007/

Park A. Artificial sweeteners and weight loss. Time Magazine.
https://time.com/collection/guide-to-weight-loss/4859012/artificial-sweeteners-weight-loss/

Trafton A. Artificial sweeteners alter gut bacteria in humans. The Scientist.
https://www.the-scientist.com/news-opinion/artificial-sweeteners-alter-gut-bacteria-in-humans-70395

Aspartame. American Cancer Society.
https://www.cancer.org/cancer/risk-prevention/chemicals/aspartame.html

Aspartame – MedlinePlus Medical Encyclopedia. MedlinePlus.
https://medlineplus.gov/ency/article/002436.htm

Saturated fats and heart disease risk. Harvard T.H. Chan School of Public Health.
https://www.hsph.harvard.edu/news/press-releases/saturated-fats-increased-heart-disease-risk/

DiNicolantonio JJ, et al. Saturated fat and cardiovascular disease: Reassessment of the evidence. Nutrients, 2023; 15(1):180.
https://www.ncbi.nlm.nih.gov/pmc/articles/PMC9794145/

What's the Difference Between Processed and Ultra-Processed Food?
https://www.healthline.com/health/food-nutrition/ultra-processed-foods

David Suzuki Foundation. "Dirty Dozen: BHA and BHT." Living Green.
https://davidsuzuki.org/living-green/dirty-dozen-bha-bht/

Loving-kindness meditation. Mindful Magazine.
https://www.mindful.org/loving-kindness-meditation-with-sharon-salzberg/

Spritzler F. What is BPA? Should I be concerned about it? Healthline, 2018.
https://www.healthline.com/nutrition/what-is-bpa

Arnold LE, Lofthouse N, Hurt E. Artificial food colors and attention-deficit/hyperactivity symptoms: conclusions to dye for. Neurotherapeutics. 2012 Jul;9(3):599-609. doi: 10.1007/s13311-012-0133-x. PMID: 22864801; PMCID: PMC3441937.

Borzelleca JF, Capen CC, Hallagan JB. Lifetime toxicity/carcinogenicity study of FD & C Red No. 3 (erythrosine) in rats. Food Chem Toxicol. 1987 Oct;25(10):723-33. doi: 10.1016/0278-6915(87)90226-2. PMID: 2824305.

Lemon & Citrus Research

Miyake T, et al. Effects of lifelong intake of lemon polyphenols on aging and intestinal microbiome in the senescence-accelerated mouse prone 1 (SAMP1). Journal of Clinical Biochemistry and Nutrition, 2019; 64(2): 122–129.
https://www.ncbi.nlm.nih.gov/pmc/articles/PMC6403313/

Nast C. 6 benefits of lemon water, explained by the experts. Vogue, 2023.
https://www.vogue.com/article/lemon-water-health-benefits

https://www.mettainstitute.org/

FOR CEREMONIAL CACAO Ora Cacao

https://ceremonial-cacao.com/

Use Code LARA81624 for 10% off

Sources for Food Holidays:

https://www.thenibble.com/fun/more/facts/food-holidays.asp

https://nationaltoday.com/food-beverage-holidays/

https://www.eatthis.com/national-food-holidays/

https://www.nationaldaycalendar.com/
https://www.usfoods.com/our-services/business-trends/let-food-holidays-work-for-you.html

NUTRITION SCHOOL and LAND OF NUTRITION

To Learn More about Institue for Integrative Nutrition, where I studied nutrition, visit https://click-myl.ink/4etu53uh
Please use my discount code if you choose to take a course: LARAMCKENNAXIIN

To learn more about working with Lara one on one, in groups, and workshops, please visit LandofNutrition.com

Acknowledgment

A big, nourishing thank you to Red Penguin Publishing for helping this dream book take shape, to my family for their endless patience and inspiration, and to my friend, Cathy, for sprinkling encouragement, early edits, and introducing me to Loving-Kindness.

Extra love to the Institute for Integrative Nutrition for fueling curiosity, and to ChatGPT for helping stir some ideas (Naughty List mostly) into shape.

All photographs and images in this book are either original or carefully chosen licensed stock.

Finally, every page of this book was created for you with love, patience, and the belief that food connects us to something greater.

Food is My Religion Recipe Index

Salads, Dressings, Sauces and Dips

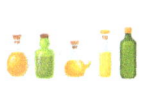 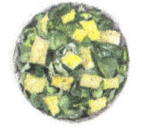 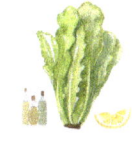 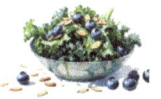 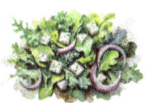

| LON Salad Dressiing | Concord Salad | Caesar Salad | Summer Salad | Yummy Kale Salad | Christmas Salad |
| Page 113 | Page 115 | Page 115 | Page 116 | Page 117 | Page 118 |

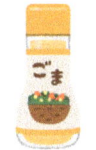 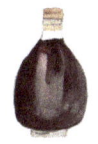 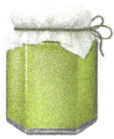 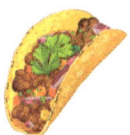 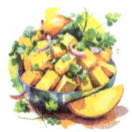 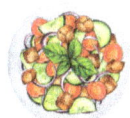

Carrot Ginger Dressing — Page 129
Asian All In One — Page 120
Chimichurri — Page 121
Taco Seasoning — Page 122
Mango Salsa — Page 123
Tzatziki & Cuc Salad — Page 124

Soups and Stews

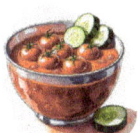 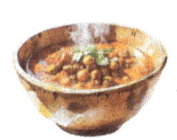 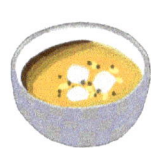 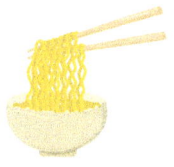 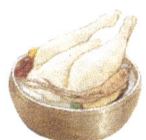

Gazpacho — Page 125
Chili - 3 ways — Page 126
Butternut Squash Soup — Page 127
Ramen Miso — Page 128
Chicken Noodle Soup — Page 130

Food is My Religion Recipe Index

Main Courses

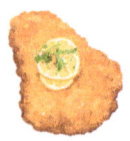 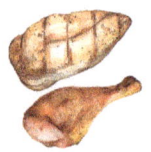 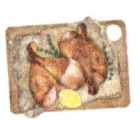 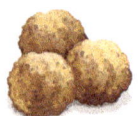 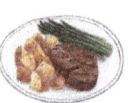 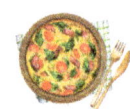

Baked Chicken Cutlet	Chicken Marinade	Lemon Chicken	Mediterranean Meatballs	Skirt Steak	Frittata
Page 132	Page 133	Page 135	Page 136	Page 137	Page 138

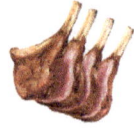 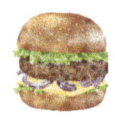 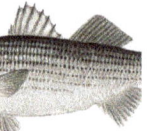 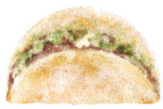  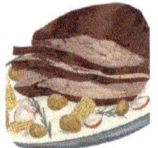

Lamb Chops	Burgers & Hot Dogs	Ceviche	TNT Tacos	Cape Cod Cod	Brisket
Page 140	Page 142	Page 144	Page 145	Page 146	Page 148

On The Side

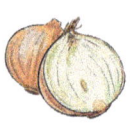 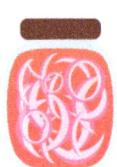 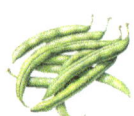 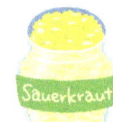 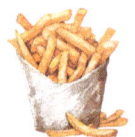 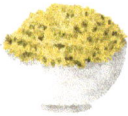

Carmelized Onion	Pickled Onion	Green Beans	Sauerkraut	French Fries	Yellow Rice
Page 149	Page 150	Page 151	Page 152	Page 154	Page 155

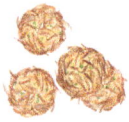 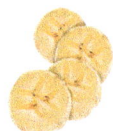

Potato Latkes	Baked Plantains
Page 156	Page 158

Part 2 Recipes

Add Something Sweet

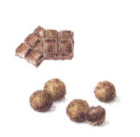
Antioxidant Truffles
Page 159

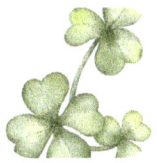
Irish Soda Bread
Page 160

Coconut Macaroons
Page 161

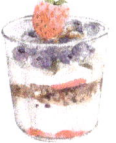
Granola
Page 162

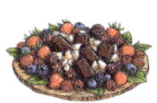
Berry Nice Boards
Page 164

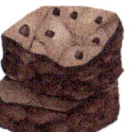
Sweet Potato Brownies
Page 165

Linzer Tarts
Page 166

Zucchini Muffins
Page 168

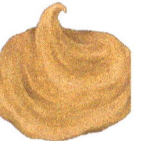
Almond Butter Chunks
Page 170

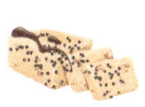
Tahini Squares
Page 171

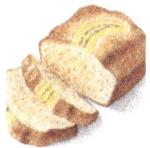
Banana Bread
Page 172

Elixers

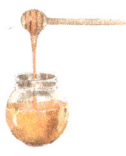
Magic Morning Tonic
Page 173

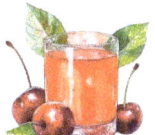
Cherry Juice Mocktail
Page 174

Thanksgiving Menu

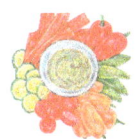
Crudités Appetizer
Page 175

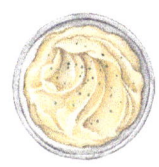
Mashed Potatoes
Page 175

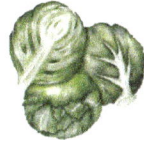
Brussel Sprouts
Page 175

Roasted Carrots
Page 175

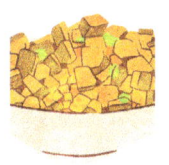
Homemade Stuffing
Page 176

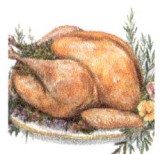
Turkey & Apple Crumb
Page 176

www.ingramcontent.com/pod-product-compliance
Lightning Source LLC
Chambersburg PA
CBHW042352070526
44585CB00028B/2899